Medifocus Guidebook on:

Ductal Carcinoma in Situ of the Breast

Last Update: 06 August 2014

Medifocus.com, Inc.

11529 Daffodil Lane
Suite 200
Silver Spring, MD 20902

www.medifocus.com

(800) 965-3002

MediFocus Guide #OC008

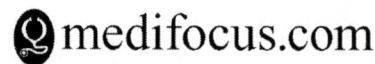

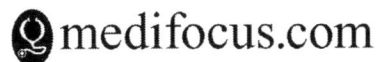

How To Use This Medifocus Guidebook

Before you start to review your *Guidebook*, it would be helpful to familiarize yourself with the organization and content of the information that is included in the Guidebook. Your *MediFocus Guidebook* is organized into the following five major sections.

- **Section 1: Background Information** - This section provides detailed information about the organization and content of the *Guidebook* including tips and suggestions for conducting additional research about the condition.

- **Section 2: The Intelligent Patient Overview** - This section is a comprehensive overview of the condition and includes important information about the cause of the disease, signs and symptoms, how the condition is diagnosed, the treatment options, quality of life issues, and questions to ask your doctor.

- **Section 3: Guide to the Medical Literature** - This section opens the door to the latest cutting-edge research and clinical advances recently published in leading medical journals. It consists of an extensive, focused selection of journal article references with links to the PubMed abstracts (summaries) of the articles. PubMed is the U.S. National Library of Medicine's database of references and abstracts from more than 4,500 medical and scientific articles published worldwide.

- **Section 4: Centers of Research** - This section is a unique directory of doctors, researchers, hospitals, medical centers, and research institutions with specialized interest and, in many cases, clinical expertise in the management of patients with the condition. You can use the "Centers of Research" directory to contact, consults, or network with leading experts in the field and to locate a hospital or medical center that can help you.

- **Section 5: Tips for Finding and Choosing a Doctor** - This section of your *Guidebook* offers important tips for how to find physicians as well as suggestions for how to make informed choices about choosing a doctor who is right for you.

- **Section 6: Directory of Organizations** - This section of your *Guidebook* is a directory of select disease organizations and support groups that are in the business of helping patients and their families by providing access to information, resources, and services. Many of these organizations can answer your questions, enable you to network with other patients, and help you find a doctor in your geographical area who specializes in managing your condition.

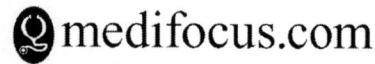

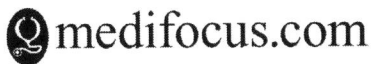

Disclaimer

Medifocus.com, Inc. serves only as a clearinghouse for medical health information and does not directly or indirectly practice medicine. Any information provided by *Medifocus.com, Inc.* is intended solely for educating our clients and should not be construed as medical advice or guidance, which should always be obtained from a licensed physician or other health-care professional. As such, the client assumes full responsibility for the appropriate use of the medical and health information contained in the Guidebook and agrees to hold *Medifocus.com, Inc.* and any of its third-party providers harmless from any and all claims or actions arising from the clients' use or reliance on the information contained in this Guidebook. Although *Medifocus.com, Inc.* makes every reasonable attempt to conduct a thorough search of the published medical literature, the possibility always exists that some significant articles may be missed.

Copyright

© Copyright 2013, *Medifocus.com, Inc.* All rights reserved as to the selection, arrangement, formatting, and presentation of the information contained in this report, including our background and introductory information.

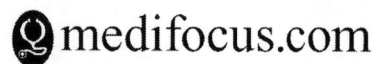

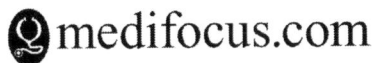

Table of Contents

Background Information 9
   Introduction 9
   About Your Medifocus Guidebook 11
   Ordering Full-Text Articles 15

The Intelligent Patient Overview 19

Guide to the Medical Literature 63
   Introduction 63
   Recent Literature: What Your Doctor Reads 65
      Review Articles 65
      General Interest Articles 78
      Drug Therapy Articles 103
      Surgical Therapy Articles 104
      Clinical Trials Articles 114
      Radiation Therapy Articles 118

Centers of Research 125
   United States 127
   Other Countries 143

Tips on Finding and Choosing a Doctor 159

Directory of Organizations 169

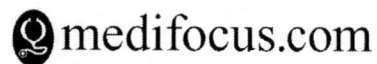

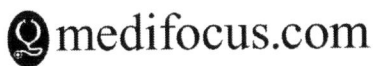

1 - Background Information

Introduction

Chronic or life-threatening illnesses can have a devastating impact on both the patient and the family. In today's new world of medicine, many consumers have come to realize that they are the ones who are primarily responsible for their own health care as well as for the health care of their loved ones.

When facing a chronic or life-threatening illness, you need to become an educated consumer in order to make an informed health care decision. Essentially that means finding out everything about the illness - the treatment options, the doctors, and the hospitals - so that you can become an educated health care consumer and make the tough decisions. In the past, consumers would go to a library and read everything available about a particular illness or medical condition. In today's world, many turn to the Internet for their medical information needs.

The first sites visited are usually the well known health "portals" or disease organizations and support groups which contain a general overview of the condition for the layperson. That's a good start but soon all of the basic information is exhausted and the need for more advanced information still exists. What are the latest "cutting-edge" treatment options? What are the results of the most up-to-date clinical trials? Who are the most notable experts? Where are the top-ranked medical institutions and hospitals?

The best source for authoritative medical information in the United States is the National Library of Medicine's medical database called PubMed, that indexes citations and abstracts (brief summaries) of over 7 million articles from more than 3,800 medical journals published worldwide. PubMed was developed for medical professionals and is the primary source utilized by health care providers for keeping up with the latest advances in clinical medicine.

A typical PubMed search for a specific disease or condition, however, usually retrieves hundreds or even thousands of "hits" of journal article citations. That's an avalanche of information that needs to be evaluated and transformed into truly useful knowledge. What are the most relevant journal articles? Which ones apply to your specific situation? Which articles are considered to be the most authoritative - the ones your physician would rely on in making clinical decisions? This is where *Medifocus.com* provides an effective solution.

Medifocus.com has developed an extensive library of *MediFocus Guidebooks* covering a wide spectrum of chronic and life threatening diseases. Each *MediFocus Guidebook* is a high quality, up- to-date digest of "professional-level" medical information consisting of the most relevant citations and abstracts of journal articles published in authoritative, trustworthy medical journals. This information represents the latest advances known to modern medicine for the treatment and management of the condition, including published results from clinical trials. Each *Guidebook* also includes a valuable index of leading authors and medical institutions as well as a directory of disease organizations and support groups. *MediFocus Guidebooks* are reviewed, revised and updated every 4-months to ensure that you receive the latest and most up-to-date information about the specific condition.

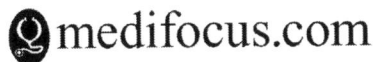

About Your MediFocus Guidebook

Introduction

Your *MediFocus Guidebook* is a valuable resource that represents a comprehensive synthesis of the most up-to-date, advanced medical information published about the condition in well-respected, trustworthy medical journals. It is the same type of professional-level information used by physicians and other health-care professionals to keep abreast of the latest developments in biomedical research and clinical medicine. The *Guidebook* is intended for patients who have a need for more advanced, in-depth medical information than is generally available to consumers from a variety of other resources. The primary goal of a *MediFocus Guidebook* is to educate patients and their families about their treatment options so that they can make informed health-care decisions and become active participants in the medical decision making process.

The *Guidebook* production process involves a team of experienced medical research professionals with vast experience in researching the published medical literature. This team approach to the development and production of the *MediFocus Guidebooks* is designed to ensure the accuracy, completeness, and clinical relevance of the information. The *Guidebook* is intended to serve as a basis for a more meaningful discussion between patients and their health-care providers in a joint effort to seek the most appropriate course of treatment for the disease.

Guidebook Organization and Content

Section 1 - Background Information
This section provides detailed information about the organization and content of the *Guidebook* including tips and suggestions for conducting additional research about the condition.

Section 2 - The Intelligent Patient Overview
This section of your *MediFocus Guidebook* represents a detailed overview of the disease or condition specifically written from the patient's perspective. It is designed to satisfy the basic informational needs of consumers and their families who are confronted with the illness and are facing difficult choices. Important aspects which are addressed in "The Intelligent Patient" section include:

- The etiology or cause of the disease
- Signs and symptoms
- How the condition is diagnosed

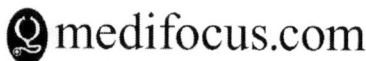

- The current standard of care for the disease
- Treatment options
- New developments
- Important questions to ask your health care provider

Section 3 - Guide to the Medical Literature

This is a roadmap to important and up-to-date medical literature published about the condition from authoritative, trustworthy medical journals. This is the same information that is used by physicians and researchers to keep up with the latest developments and breakthroughs in clinical medicine and biomedical research. A broad spectrum of articles is included in each *MediFocus Guidebook* to provide information about standard treatments, treatment options, new clinical developments, and advances in research. To facilitate your review and analysis of this information, the articles are grouped by specific categories. A typical *MediFocus Guidebook* usually contains one or more of the following article groupings:

- *Review Articles:* Articles included in this category are broad in scope and are intended to provide the reader with a detailed overview of the condition including such important aspects as its cause, diagnosis, treatment, and new advances.

- *General Interest Articles:* These articles are broad in scope and contain supplementary information about the condition that may be of interest to select groups of patients.

- *Drug Therapy:* Articles that provide information about the effectiveness of specific drugs or other biological agents for the treatment of the condition.

- *Surgical Therapy:* Articles that provide information about specific surgical treatments for the condition.

- *Clinical Trials:* Articles in this category summarize studies which compare the safety and efficacy of a new, experimental treatment modality to currently available standard treatments for the condition. In many cases, clinical trials represent the latest advances in the field and may be considered as being on the "cutting edge" of medicine. Some of these experimental treatments may have already been incorporated into clinical practice.

The following information is provided for each of the articles referenced in this section of your *MediFocus Guidebook:*

- Article title

- Author Name(s)
- Institution where the study was done
- Journal reference (Volume, page numbers, year of publication)
- Link to Abstract (brief summary of the actual article)

Linking to Abstracts: Most of the medical journal articles referenced in this section of your *MediFocus Guidebook* include an abstract (brief summary of the actual article) that can be accessed online via the National Library of Medicine's PubMed® database. You can easily access the individual article abstracts online by entering the individual URL address for a particular article into your web browser, or by going to the URL listed on the bottom of each page of this section.

Section 4 - Centers of Research

We've compiled a unique directory of doctors, researchers, medical centers, and research institutions with specialized research interest, and in many cases, clinical expertise in the management of the specific medical condition. The "Centers of Research" directory is a valuable resource for quickly identifying and locating leading medical authorities and medical institutions within the United States and other countries that are considered to be at the forefront in clinical research and treatment of the condition.

Inclusion of the names of specific doctors, researchers, hospitals, medical centers, or research institutions in this *Guidebook* does not imply endorsement by Medifocus.com, Inc. or any of its affiliates. Consumers are encouraged to conduct additional research to identify health-care professionals, hospitals, and medical institutions with expertise in providing specific medical advice, guidance, and treatment for this condition.

Section 5 - Tips on Finding and Choosing a Doctor

One of the most important decisions confronting patients who have been diagnosed with a serious medical condition is finding and choosing a qualified physician who will deliver high-level, quality medical care in accordance with curently accepted guidelines and standards of care. Finding the "best" doctor to manage your condition, however, can be a frustrating and time-consuming experience unless you know what you are looking for and how to go about finding it. This section of your Guidebook offers important tips for how to find physicians as well as suggestions for how to make informed choices about choosing a doctor who is right for you.

Section 6 - Directory of Organizations

This section of your *Guidebook* is a directory of select disease organizations and support groups that are in the business of helping patients and their families by providing access to information, resources, and services. Many of these organizations can answer your questions, enable you to network with other patients, and help you find a doctor in your

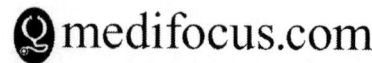

geographical area who specializes in managing your condition.

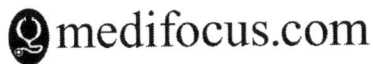

Ordering Full-Text Articles

After reviewing your *MediFocus Guidebook*, you may wish to order the full-text copy of some of the journal article citations that are referenced in the *Guidebook*. There are several options available for obtaining full-text copies of journal articles, however, with the exception of obtaining the article yourself by visiting a nearby medical library, most involve a fee to cover the costs of photocopying, delivering, and paying the copyright royalty fees set by the individual publishers of medical journals.

This section of your *MediFocus Guidebook* provides some basic information about how you can go about obtaining full-text copies of journal articles from various fee-based document delivery resources.

Commercial Document Delivery Services

There are numerous commercial document delivery companies that provide full-text photocopying and delivery services to the general public. The costs may vary from company to company so it is worth your while to carefully shop-around and compare prices. Some of these commercial document delivery services enable you to order articles directly online from the company's web site. You can locate companies that provide document delivery services by typing the key words "document delivery" into any major Internet search engine.

National Library of Medicine's "Loansome Doc" Document Retrieval Services

The National Library of Medicine (NLM), located in Bethesda, Maryland, offers full-text photocopying and delivery of journal articles through its on-line service known as "Loansome Doc". To learn more about how you can order articles using "Loansome Doc", please visit the NLM web site at:
http://www.nlm.nih.gov/pubs/factsheets/loansome_doc.html

Participating "Loansome Doc" Libraries: United States

In the United States there are approximately 250 medical libraries that participate in the National Library of Medicine's "Loansome Doc" document retrieval and delivery services for the general public. Please note that each participating library sets its own policies and

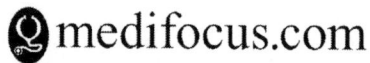

charges for providing document retrieval services. To order full-text copies of articles, simply contact a participating "Loansome Doc" medical library in your geographical area and ask to speak with one of the reference librarians. They can answer all of your questions including fees, delivery options, and turn-around time.

Here is how to find a participating "Loansome Doc" library in the U.S. that provides article retrieval services for the general public:

- **United States** - Contact a Regional Medical Library at 1-800-338-7657 (Monday - Friday; 8:30 AM - 5:30 PM). They will provide information about libraries in your area with which you may establish an account for the "Loansome Doc" service.

- **Canada** - Contact the Canada Institute for Scientific and Technical Information (CISTI) at 1-800-668-1222 for information about libraries in your area.

International MEDLARS Centers

If you reside outside the United States, you can obtain copies of medical journal articles through one of several participating International Medical Literature Analysis and Retrieval Systems (MEDLARS) Centers that provide "Loansome Doc" services in over 20 major countries. International MEDLARS Centers can be found in some of these countries: Australia, Canada, China, Egypt, France, Germany, Hong Kong, India, Israel, Italy, Japan, Korea, Kuwait, Mexico, Norway, Russia, South Africa, Sweden, and the United Kingdom. A complete listing of International MEDLARS Centers, including locations and telephone contact information can be viewed at:
http://www.nlm.nih.gov/pubs/factsheets/intlmedlars.html

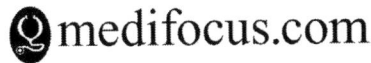

NOTES

Use this page for taking notes as you review your Guidebook

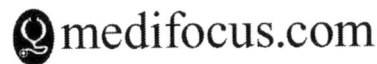

2 - The Intelligent Patient Overview

DUCTAL CARCINOMA IN SITU OF THE BREAST

Introduction to Ductal Carcinoma in Situ

The female breast is made up of glands that produce and release milk after childbirth. The glands that make the milk are called *lobules* and the tubes that connect them to the nipple are called *ducts*. The breast itself is made up of lobules, ducts, and fatty, connective, and lymphatic tissue.

Lymph is a clear fluid that contains immune system cells. The fluid is carried in *lymphatic vessels* that lead to small, pea-sized collections of tissue called *lymph nodes*. Most lymphatic vessels of the breast lead to lymph nodes under the arm called *axillary lymph nodes*.

There are several types of tumors that can occur in the breasts. Most are benign (non-cancerous) and are related to fibrocystic changes. Cysts are fluid-filled sacs and fibrosis refers to the forming of connective tissue or scar tissue. Benign breast tumors are abnormal growths, but they do not appear outside of the breast and they are not life threatening.

Breast cancer is the most common cancer among women, other than skin cancer. It is the second leading cause of cancer death in women after lung cancer. Fortunately, deaths from breast cancer have declined significantly, which is though to be due to better detection and improved treatment.

Ductal carcinoma in situ (DCIS) of the breast is an early, localized cluster of cancer cells that start in the milk passages (ducts) but have not penetrated the duct walls into the surrounding tissue. The term "in situ" refers to a tumor that has not spread beyond the place where it originally developed. By definition, DCIS is a non-invasive form of breast cancer because the cancer cells are confined to the milk ducts of the breast.

Ductal carcinoma in situ is sometimes described as "pre-cancerous", "pre-invasive", "non-invasive", or "intraductal carcinoma". Although, by definition, DCIS is a non-invasive form of breast cancer, if left untreated, it may progress to 'true' breast cancer

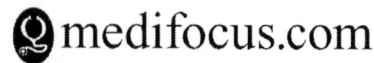

by spreading into and invading the surrounding healthy breast tissue. Because doctors cannot predict with any degree of certainty whether DCIS will develop into invasive breast cancer, early diagnosis and treatment is crucial. With appropriate treatment, the prognosis (outlook) for women with DCIS is excellent.

Fortunately, DCIS can often be detected on screening mammography before any symptoms develop. Ductal carcinoma in situ usually appears on mammography as an area of *microcalcification* (groups of small calcifications clustered together within the breast). With the increased availability of mammography, breast cancers are being detected earlier.

The incidence of DCIS has increased dramatically since the introduction of widespread screening mammography. In 1983, approximately 5,000 cases of DCIS were reported, however, due to the widespread use of screening mammography, the number of women being diagnosed with DCIS has increased about 10-fold. According to the American Cancer Society, approximately 54,000 cases of DCIS were diagnosed in the United States in 2010.

According to a study published in January 2010 in the *Journal of the National Cancer Institute*, the incidence of DCIS in the United States has increased from 1.87 per 100,000 during 1973 - 1975 to 32.5 per 100,000 in 2004. Although an increase in the incidence of DCIS was found across all age groups, the greatest increase in incidence of DCIS was found in women over age 50. According to this study, approximately 15% of women diagnosed with DCIS and treated with either lumpectomy or mastectomy later went on to develop invasive breast cancer.

Ductal carcinoma in situ represents 10-15% of all new breast cancers diagnosed in the United States and accounts for 30-50% of cancers detected by screening mammography in women less than age 50 and 15-25% in women over age 50. It also comprises approximately 7-10% of all breast biopsies.

Fortunately, DCIS is a highly curable disease with a 10-year cancer-specific survival of about 97%. Because DCIS is a "forerunner" of invasive breast cancer, early diagnosis and treatment are crucial for reducing the risk of developing invasive breast cancer.

Most Common Types of Breast Cancer

The most common types of breast cancers are *adenocarcinomas* that originate in the ducts or lobules of the breast. There are two main types of breast adenocarcinomas known as *ductal carcinomas* and *lobular carcinomas*. These can further be divided into the following subtypes:

- Ductal carcinoma in situ (DCIS)

    - represents the most common form of noninvasive breast cancer
    - may contain areas of necrotic (dead) cancer cells
    - pathologists use the term *comedocarcinoma* or *comedo DCIC* to describe DCIS if necrotic cancer cells are observed under a microscope
    - comedo DCIS is considered to be a more aggressive type of disease than non-comedo DCIS

- Lobular carcinoma in situ (LCIS)

    - LCIS is also considered to represent a noninvasive form of breast cancer
    - LCIS starts in the milk-producing lobules of the breast but does not penetrate the walls of the lobules.
    - the term "in situ" in the term "lobular carcinoma in situ" indicates that this is an early stage of breast cancer that is confined locally to area where the cancer started
    - some doctors believe that LCIS is a risk factor for developing invasive breast cancer and women with LCIS should undergo a physical exam at least twice each year as well as a yearly mammogram.

- Infiltrating (invasive) ductal carcinoma (IDC)

    - IDC is the most common type of breast cancer and represents about 80% of all invasive breast cancers.
    - IDC starts in the ducts of the breast but spreads to invade the surrounding normal breast tissue.

- Infiltrating (invasive) lobular carcinoma (ILC)

    - ILC is also considered as an invasive form of breast cancer but is much less common than IDC.
    - ILC starts in the lobules of the breast but can spread (metastasize) to other parts of the body.
    - ILC may be more difficult to detect with screening mammography than IDC.

Stages of Breast Cancer

Staging is the process of assessing how far the cancer has spread and is important in making treatment decisions and determining prognosis.

- Stage 0 - Noninvasive, Carcinoma in situ (DCIS)

- Stage I - Cancer cells have not spread beyond the breast and the tumor is no more than about an inch (2.5 cm or less) across

- Stage II - The tumor in the breast is less than 1 inch across and the cancer has spread to the lymph nodes under the arm, OR

    - the tumor is between 1 and 2 inches (less than 5.0 cm) with or without spread to the lymph nodes under the arm, OR
    - the tumor is larger than 2 inches (more than 5.0 cm) but has not spread to the lymph nodes under the arm

- Stage III - "Locally advanced cancer" - The tumor in the breast is large (more than 2 inches across) and the cancer is extensive in the underarm lymph nodes or It has spread to other lymph nodes or tissues near the breast. This stage includes inflammatory breast cancer.

- Stage IV - The cancer is metastatic, meaning it has spread from the breast to other parts of body.

Recurrent breast cancer means the disease has recurred despite initial treatment. Most recurrences appear within the first 2 or 3 years but can occur many years later.

Classification of Ductal Carcinoma in Situ

Ductal carcinoma in situ (DCIS) of the breast is not a single disease but rather a diversified group of breast lesions. Various types of DCIS can be distinguished on the basis of histological features, genetic characteristics, clinical symptoms, and radiographic appearance on mammography. Consequently, the biological behavior of different types of DCIS is also highly diversified. Although DCIS has the potential to develop into invasive breast cancer, the risk of malignant potential varies widely among the different types of DCIS. Clearly, most types of DCIS do not progress to invasive breast cancer, however, the fact that some evolve into malignant breast cancer indicates that they are more "aggressive" from a biological perspective. Unfortunately, at the present time, doctors cannot predict with absolute certainty which types of DCIS will eventually progress to invasive breast cancer.

In order to better estimate the malignant potential of DCIS, several different classification systems have been developed. It is important to note, however, that most of these classification systems more accurately predict the likelihood of recurrence of DCIS after surgical excision of the initial tumor rather than the likelihood for DCIS to progress to invasive breast cancer.

The traditional classification method for DCIS is based upon the appearance of the cells when examined under a microscope (histological features). Several histological parameters can be used to distinguish and classify the different types of DCIS. One classification scheme is based upon the presence or absence of necrotic (dead) cells at the center of the breast ducts. According to this classification system, DCIS may be grouped as follows:

- *Comedo DCIS* - characterized by the presence of necrotic (dead) cells at the center of the breast ducts (comedonecrosis). The comedo type of DCIS is usually a more aggressive than the non-comedo type of DCIS (absence of necrotic cells).

- *Non-comedo* types of DCIS include:
    - Micropapillary DCIS
    - Cribiform DCIS
    - Solid DCIS
    - Papillary DCIS

Another important histological parameter that can be used to classify DCIS is *nuclear grade* - an evaluation of the size and shape of the nucleus in the tumor cells and the percentage of tumor cells that are in the process of dividing and growing. On the basis of nuclear grade, DCIS can be classified into one of the following three groups:

- Low-nuclear-grade DCIS
- Intermediate-nuclear-grade DCIS
- High-nuclear-grade DCIS

Nuclear grade has been found to be an important feature that helps doctors predict the likelihood of recurrence of DCIS after surgery. In an article published in 2003 in the *Journal of the National Cancer Institute*, researchers from the San Francisco Veterans Affairs Medical Center conducted a study of 1,036 women age 40 or older who were diagnosed with DCIS and treated with *lumpectomy* (surgical removal of a tumor and a small amount of surrounding tissue). The researchers reported that women with high-nuclear-grade DCIS had a 5-year risk of an invasive recurrence of 11.8% compared to only 4.8% for women with low-nuclear-grade DCIS. The finding that women with high-nuclear-grade DCIS are about 2.5 times more likely to develop an invasive recurrence than women with low-nuclear-grade DCIS, indicates that they should undergo additional treatment, such as postoperative radiation therapy, in order to reduce the risk of invasive recurrence. As mentioned previously, comedonecrosis (the presence of dead cells at the center of the breast ducts) is another histological feature that carries a high risk of invasive recurrence because comedo DCIS is usually associated with a high-nuclear grade.

In 1996, another classification system called the Van Nuys prognostic index (VNPI) was introduced to help doctors more accurately predict the risk of local recurrence after surgical excision of DCIS. The VNPI is a tool that uses the following four variables (prognostic indicators) to predict the likelihood of recurrence of DCIS in women following breast-conserving surgery:

- Tumor size
- Margin width
- Nuclear grade
- Comedonecrosis (present or absent)

In 2003, the VNPI was modified to include a woman's age as an additional prognostic indicator since younger age has been found to be associated with a higher risk of recurrence of DCIS.

A newer classification system for DCIS was proposed in 2006 that takes into account both histological features as well as molecular features in order to better predict the malignant potential of DCIS. Researchers have found that certain molecular abnormalities are associated with a more aggressive type of DCIS that increases its likelihood for developing into invasive breast cancer. Examples of some molecular features that are associated with more aggessive tumors include:

- Mutation of a gene called p53 (located on chromosome #17) that produces a protein called the p53 tumor suppressive protein. A tumor suppressive protein helps to prevent the uncontrolled proliferation and growth of cells. Mutation of the p53 gene leads to the production of a defective p53 tumor suppressive protein which cannot act to suppress the proliferation and growth of cells, thereby leading to cancer.

- Overexpression (amplification) of a human growth factor receptor called C-erbB2.

- Overexpression of a cellular molecular marker of proliferation called Ki-67.

In this classification system, DCIS is classified as either "highly aggressive"; "moderately aggressive"; or "low aggressive" using a combination of histological features (e.g., comedonecrosis, nuclear grade) and molecular abnormalities (e.g., p53; C-erbB2; Ki-67).

Doctors can use this classification system to make better treatment decisions for women with DCIS. For example, since "highly aggressive" DCIS has the greatest postential for local recurrence within 2 years after surgical excision and for progression to invasive breast cancer within 5 to 10 years, women with "highly agressive" DCIS should be treated either by mastectomy or by local excision plus radiation therapy and, possibly, hormonal therapy. Women with "low aggressive" DCIS, on the other hand, can theoretically be treated with simple local excision alone since the risk of local recurrence and progression to invasive breast cancer is much lower.

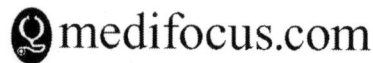

Diagnosis of Ductal Carcinoma in Situ

Clinical Evaluation of Ductal Carcinoma in Situ

The initial steps in the diagnostic "work-up" of a patient with suspected ductal carcinoma in situ (DCIS) involve a careful history and physical examination. In the past, before the widespread use of screening mammography, most patients with DCIS presented to their doctor with a breast mass or lump that was large enough to be felt or palpated (palpable breast mass) or with nipple discharge. Since the 1980's, when screening mammography became more widely available, most women with DCIS have no clinical signs or symptoms of breast disease and only a small percentage present with a palpable breast mass or nipple discharge.

Signs and Symptoms of Ductal Carcinoma in Situ

In the past, most women with ductal carcinoma in situ (DCIS) had a mass large enough to be felt (the average size of a DCIS mass discovered on exam was 60 mm) or nipple discharge before the diagnosis could be made. Since screening mammography became more widely available in the 1980s, many cases of DCIS are discovered before any symptoms develop and the average size of DCIS has been reduced to 10 mm at the time of discovery. It has been estimated that DCIS accounts for about 20% of all mammographically detected breast cancers.

In general, signs and symptoms of breast cancer may include:

- Lump or mass felt in the breast or under the arm
- Recent changes in the appearance of the nipple (i.e., inversion or retraction)
- Dimpling or "orange peel" appearance of the breast
- New asymmetry of the breasts (a change in the contour of the breast where one breast is higher than the other)
- Nipple discharge that is bloody or foul smelling - Nipple discharge is not always a symptom of breast cancer. Spontaneous nipple discharge is associated with carcinoma about 20-25% of the time. Expressed nipple discharge is usually due to medication or hormonal causes.

Mammographic Evaluation of Ductal Carcinoma in Situ

To date, mammography is the most effective imaging modality for detecting ductal carcinoma in situ (DCIS) and plays an important role in determining various details about the mass, including:

- Microcalcification is the most common feature of DCIS that is observed by mammography.
- Microcalcification is an area where tiny specks of calcium have formed in the ducts of the breast.
- It has been estimated that up to 90% of patients with DCIS have microcalcification that is evident by mammography.
- Mammography is also used to estimate the size of the DCIS which is an important factor in the surgical decision-making process. Unfortunately, mammography is not completely accurate for estimating the size of the DCIS and may underestimate the actual size of the lesion.
- In cases where DCIS is detected in one breast, the other breast is also examined by mammography since approximately 10 to 20% of women with DCIS have lesions in both breasts.

The role of other imaging modalities such as *magnetic resonance imaging* (MRI) and *breast ultrasonography* in diagnosing and staging DCIS have not been established and, therefore, these imaging techniques are not routinely employed.

Diagnostic Biopsy for Ductal Carcinoma in Situ

When an abnormal area has been detected by mammography and ductal carcinoma in situ (DCIS) is suspected, the diagnosis must be confirmed by removing a sample from the suspicious area of the breast and examining the specimen under a microscope. This procedure is known as a *diagnostic biopsy*.

Traditionally, most cases of mammographically detected nonpalpable DCIS have been diagnosed by a procedure known as *wire-localization open surgical biopsy*. This procedure is usually performed on an "outpatient" basis in the Radiology department of the hospital or surgical center where your breast biopsy is scheduled. After numbing the breast with a local anesthetic, the doctor will insert a very fine needle into the area of the breast that appeared to be abnormal on the mammogram. Once the needle has been inserted into the target area, a slender wire is threaded through the needle until it reaches the target area. The needle is then removed and another mammogram is taken to verify that the wire is in the proper location. Your surgeon will then perform a breast biopsy during which the wire is removed and tissue from the suspicious area is removed for examination under a microscope.

Recently, a more accurate diagnostic biopsy technique for women with suspected DCIS has been developed called *directional vacuum-assisted biopsy* (DVAB). Currently, there are three types of DVAB systems available commercially:

- Mammotome
- Spirotome
- Minimally Invasive Breast Biopsy (MIBB)

For the DVAB procedure, which is also performed in an "outpatient" setting, the breast is numbed with a local anesthetic and a small incision is created through which the surgeon inserts the DVAB device (a hollow probe) and, using stereotactic-guidance, advances the device into the abnormal area of breast tissue. DVAB devices use a vacuum (suction) to pull tissue into the hollow probe and the tissue is cut with a rotating knife that is attached to the probe. Using the DVAB device, the surgeon can remove several pieces of tissue from the abnormal area of the breast without having to withdraw the device each time. The DVAB device reduces the risk of sampling error and is, therefore, considered a more accurate breast biopsy technique as compared to the traditional *core-needle biopsy*.

A breast biopsy for suspected DCIS should be performed by a qualified surgeon and patients should not hesitate to ask the doctor about their training and experience with this procedure prior to consenting to undergo a breast biopsy.

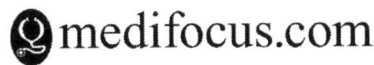

Treatment Options for Ductal Carcinoma in Situ

Goals of Treatment for Ductal Carcinoma in Situ

If ductal carcinoma in situ (DCIS) is left untreated, the cells may invade the surrounding breast tissue and may spread via the lymph nodes to other areas of the body (invasive cancer). Long-term follow-up studies of women with **untreated DCIS** have shown that a significant number (between 15 to 60%) developed invasive breast cancer usually within 10-years.

The primary goals of treatment of DCIS is prevention of local recurrence and invasive breast cancer. When breast-conserving surgery is appropriate, the goals of treatment include the total surgical removal of the DCIS with minimal cosmetic deformity.

Current treatment options for women with DCIS include:

- Surgery alone (mastectomy or breast-conserving surgery)
- Breast-conserving surgery followed by radiation therapy
- Breast-conserving surgery followed by radiation therapy and hormonal therapy.

Surgery for Ductal Carcinoma in Situ

The surgical treatment options for women with ductal carcinoma in situ (DCIS) include:

- Simple mastectomy - surgical removal of a breast leaving the underlying muscles and lymph nodes intact.
- Breast-conserving surgery - during breast conserving surgery (also known as a *lumpectomy*), the tumor is surgically removed while leaving the remaining breast tissues, nipple, and areola intact.

Historically, DCIS was treated with mastectomy while breast-conserving surgery is a more recent treatment option for women with DCIS. Mastectomy is a curative treatment for approximately 98% of women with DCIS. Although the rates of local or regional recurrence are much lower after mastectomy as compared to breast-conserving surgery, there does not appear to be any significant differences in terms of survival between these two surgical treatment options for patients with DCIS. Breast cancer related deaths 10-years after the diagnosis of DCIS is only 1% to 2 % regardless of the type of surgery (mastectomy or lumpectomy) employed.

Mastectomy may be recommended by your surgeon as the surgical treatment of choice in certain situations. Examples include:

- If large areas of DCIS are present that cannot be surgically removed while preserving the cosmetic appearance of the breast.

- If multiple areas of DCIS are present in the same breast that cannot be removed by a single incision.

- If the patient is not considered a good candidate for postoperative radiation therapy. This includes:

  - patients who have undergone previous radiation therapy to the breast or chest area.
  - patients with an underlying connective tissue disease disorder (e.g., scleroderma, systemic lupus erythemotosus).
  - patients who are pregnant at the time that radiation therapy would be necessary.

- Women with small breasts in whom it may not be possible to achieve a good cosmetic outcome following local excision of a significant amount of breast tissue.

- Women who develop a recurrence of DCIS after initial local excision where additional local resections would result in significant breast deformity.

- Women who may prefer a mastectomy in order to avoid the inconveniences associated with postoperative radiation therapy that would be necessary following breast-conserving surgery.

As noted previously, most women who are diagnosed with DCIS by screening mammography have no clinical symptoms of the disease (such as a palpable breast mass). Because most DCIS lesions that are detected mammographically are small, there has been a shift in recent years from mastectomy to breast-conserving surgery. In fact, at the present time, in the United States most women with DCIS are treated with breast-conserving surgery.

A newer type of mastectomy procedure, known as a *skin-sparing mastectomy*, may be a reasonable option for women with DCIS since it achieves a better cosmetic outcome as compared to a simple (total) mastectomy. With a skin-sparing mastectomy, the surgeon creates a much smaller incision (called a "keyhole" incision) around the *areola*. Although the same amount of breast tissue is removed as with a simple (total) mastectomy, because the incision is smaller, 90% of the skin is preserved and scarring is usually minimal. Breast reconstruction is usually performed immediately after a skin-sparing mastectomy using tissue from the patient's abdomen or a muscle in the back called the *latissimus dorsi*.

Irrespective of whether DCIS is treated by mastectomy or breast-conserving surgery, dissection of the axillary lymph nodes (the lymph nodes located under the armpit) is not routinely indicated in patients with DCIS. This is because the risk of metastases (spread) of DCIS to the axillary lymph nodes is less than 5% and recent research has demonstrated that the risk of axillary metastases is even lower for patients with small, mammographically detected DCIS.

The role of *sentinel lymph node biopsy* and mapping in the management of patients with DCIS has recently been the subject of considerable discussion in the medical literature. Sentinel lymph node biopsy is a procedure whereby a radioactive substance, called a "tracer" is injected around the tumor site. Following injection of the tracer, a blue dye is also injected around the tumor site. The radioactive tracer and the dye are carried by the lymph fluid to the first lymph node, called the *sentinel lymph node*, that drains lymph from the tumor. The sentinel lymph node is the primary lymph node that is most likely to contain cancer cells if the tumor has metastasized from the breast. In general, routine sentinel lymph node biopsy and mapping is not currently advocated for most patients with DCIS. The main indications for this procedure include:

- Patients with high-nuclear-grade DCIS who are at the highest risk for developing invasive cancer.

- Patients with clinical symptoms of DCIS, such as a palpable breast mass.

- Patients with DCIS who require a mastectomy since this procedure cannot be performed after a mastectomy in the event that the tumor has spread to the lymph nodes.

A study published in the April 5, 2012 issue of the *Journal of the National Cancer Institute* underscored that women with DCIS who opt for breast-conserving surgery (BCS) need to understand that this choice carries with it the possibility of additional diagnostic and invasive procedures in the treated breast over several years of follow-up. The study reported that of nearly 3,000 women with DCIS who chose BCS over mastectomy, 31% underwent one or more diagnostic mammograms, and 62% had one or more invasive diagnostic procedures in the same breast during follow-up. The authors of the study concluded that since women undergoing BCS for DCIS are likely to have diagnostic and invasive procedures in the conserved breast over an extended period of time, this fact should be taken into consideration in discussions about treatment options.

Radiation Therapy for Ductal Carcinoma in Situ

Because women who undergo breast-conserving surgery for ductal carcinoma in situ (DCIS) are at risk for recurrence of a tumor (invasive or in situ) either in the same or contralateral breast, radiation therapy (radiotherapy) may be used to treat the remaining breast tissue. Most commonly, radiation therapy is used in cases of high-grade DCIS. Radiotherapy is usually given daily for 3 to 6 weeks.

Research has shown that radiation therapy following breast-conserving surgery for DCIS reduces the risk of recurrence in the same breast by up-to 50%. In the United States, the current practice is to administer radiation therapy following breast-conserving surgery for DCIS to prevent recurrence.

Currently, research is focusing on identifying subpopulations of women with DCIS who may not require radiation therapy after breast-conserving surgery. The most likely candidates for omitting radiation therapy would be women with small DCIS lesions, especially those with low- or intermediate-grade DCIS.

In an article published in 2009 in the *Journal of Clinical Oncology* (Volume 27; pp. 5319-5324), investigators from the Eastern Cooperative Oncology Group and the North Central Cancer Treatment Group reported the results of a multicenter clinical trial in which they evaluated the risk of tumor recurrence and overall survival in women with DCIS who underwent breast-conserving surgery without radiation therapy. The study population consisted of 670 women with nonpalpable DCIS who were considered suitable for breast-conserving surgery. The women who were enrolled in the study were stratified into the following two cohorts:

- Group #1 - 565 women with low- or intermediate-grade DCIS where size of the tumor was 2.5 cm or smaller. The median patient age for this group was 60 years (range = 28 to 88 years).
- Group #2 - 105 women with high-grade DCIS where the size of the tumor was 1.0 cm or smaller. The median patient age for this group was 59 years (range = 33 to 87 years).

All of the women who were enrolled in the study, which was conducted from 1997 to 2002, were treated with breast-conserving surgery without radiation therapy. Women who were enrolled into the study after 2000 were also given the option to receive adjuvant hormonal therapy with tamoxifen if their DCIS tumor was found to be estrogen-receptor positive. The median follow-up for all patients included in the study was 6.3 years during which time the investigators evaluated the number of ipsilateral breast events (IBE's). An

IBE was defined as the occurence of either invasive cancer or DCIS in the same breast that had been treated with breast-conserving surgery. The number of contralateral breast events (tumors occurring in the opposite breast) was also recorded.

The major findings of the study can be summarized as follows:

- Incidence of ipsilateral breast events (IBE's):

  - Group #1 - A total of 49 IBE's were recorded in this group of which 53% were invasive breast cancer and 47% were DCIS only. The 5-year rate of IBE's in this group was 6.1%.
  - Group #2 - A total of 17 IBE's were recorded among this group of which 35% were invasive cancer and 65% were DCIS only. The 5-year rate of IBE's in this group was 15.3%.

- Incidence of contralateral breast events:

  - Group #1 - A total of 23 contralateral breast events occurred in this group of which 65% were invasive cancer and 35% were DCIS only.
  - Group #2 - A total of 6 contralateral breast events occurred in this group all of which were invasive breast cancer.

- Women who developed a recurrence of DCIS only were treated with either breast-conserving surgery or mastectomy. Those women who developed invasive breast cancer were treated with surgery and chemotherapy.
- The overall 5-year survival rates of the two groups were as follows:

  - Group #1 - 96%
  - Group #2 - 97%

- A total of 46 patients died during the course of the study, however, none of these deaths occurred as a result of breast cancer

In summary, this multicenter clinical trial has demonstrated that breast-conserving surgery without radiation therapy may be suitable for select patients with low- or intermediate-grade DCIS measuring 2.5 cm or smaller. The 5-year rate of ipsilateral breast events (IBE's) of 6.1% in this group of women was relatively low. In contrast, women in this study with high-grade DCIS had a much higher incidence of IBE's (15.3%), suggesting that breast-conserving surgery alone without follow-up radiation therapy is inadequate treatment for these patients. Currently, the practice in the United States is to administer radiation therapy to all women with DCIS who elect to undergo breast-conserving surgery. Perhaps this practice may change in the near as more data becomes available through

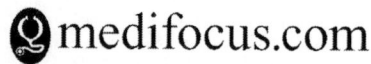

additional research regarding the risks and benefits of omitting radiation therapy after breast-conserving surgery in women with DCIS.

Adjuvant Hormonal Therapy for Ductal Carcinoma in Situ

Tamoxifen is an anti-hormone drug that belongs to a class of pharmacological agents known as selective *estrogen receptor modulators*. Tamoxifen is used for the treatment of certain types of breast cancers that are hormone sensitive. In some women with ductal carcinoma in situ (DCIS), the cancer cells contain (express) estrogen receptors on their surface. Doctors refer to this type of DCIS as "estrogen receptor positive DCIS". This means that when these cancer cells are exposed to estrogen, a naturally occurring female sex hormone, the estrogen binds to the estrogen receptor on the surface of the cells and causes them to actively grow and divide. Tomoxifen counteracts the effects of estrogen by binding to the estrogen receptors on the surface of the estrogen receptor positive breast cancer cells and, thereby, blocking estrogen from binding to the cells and preventing them from growing and dividing.

Tamoxifen is sometimes used as *adjuvant therapy* (a treatment that improves the outcome of a primary therapy) in women with DCIS who have undergone breast-conserving surgery and radiation therapy. The results of the National Surgical Adjuvant Breast and Bowel Project (NSABP) demonstrated that tomoxifen reduced the likelihood of recurrence of DCIS in the same breast as well the risk of a tumor developing in the contralateral (opposite) breast.

Currently, in the United States, adjuvant hormonal therapy with tamoxifen is recommended for select women with DCIS who undergo breast-conserving surgery. Patients who are considered as good candidates for adjuvant tamoxifen therapy include:

- Women with estrogen-receptor positive DCIS (about 75% of women with DCIS are estrogen-receptor positive).

- Younger women

- Women without risk factors for the potential side-effects of tamoxifen (previous history of stroke or pulmonary embolism)

Since its initial approval by the U.S. Food and Drug Administration in 1977, tamoxifen has been found to:

- Lower the risk of recurrence and death in women with early-stage, hormone receptor positive breast cancer

- Reduce the risk of invasive breast cancer following breast-conserving surgery in women with DCIS

- Reduce the risk of breast cancer in high-risk women

In June, 2002 the U.S. Food and Drug Administration and Astra Zeneca added a boxed warning and strengthened the "WARNINGS" section of the label for Nolvadex (tomoxifen citrate) to inform healthcare professionals about new risk information of particular relevance to women with DCIS and women at high risk for developing breast cancer and are receiving or considering Nolvadex therapy to reduce their risk of developing invasive breast cancer. Serious, life-threatening or fatal events associated with Nolvadex in the risk reduction setting (women at high risk for cancer and women with DCIS) include endometrial cancer, uterine sarcoma, stroke, and pulmonary embolism. Healthcare providers should discuss the potential benefits versus the potential risks of these serious events with women considering Nolvadex to reduce their risk of developing breast cancer.

Because of the potentially serious side-effects associated with tamoxifen therapy, researchers are currently investigating the feasibility of alternative drugs to prevent local recurrence and/or invasive breast cancer in women with DCIS after breast-conserving surgery. One class of drugs currently under investigation is known as *aromatose inhibitors*. Examples of aromatase inhibitors include ansatrozole (Arimidex) and letrozole (Femara). Currently, the role of aromatose inhibitors in the management of patients with DCIS is limited to clinical trials and tamoxifen remains as the drug of choice for adjuvant hormonal therapy.

Recurrence of Ductal Carcinoma in Situ

The rate of tumor recurrence in women with ductal carcinoma in situ (DCIS) has been estimated as approximately 0.5% to 1% per year. Although research suggests that the rates of local or regional recurrence are significantly lower after mastectomy than after breast-conserving surgery, the 10-year survival rate is approximately 98% with each of these surgical procedures.

Risk factors for tumor recurrence after breast-conserving surgery for DCIS include:

- Positive Surgical Margins - With DCIS, the pathologist examining the tissue samples removed at the time of surgery looks carefully to determine the presence of any

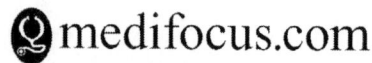

cancer cells in the margins surrounding the site of the tumor. If cancer cells are detected at the margins of the tumor, there is an increased risk of recurrence following breast-conserving surgery.

- Type of DCIS - High-grade DCIS and comedonecrosis DCIS lesions are associated with an increased risk of local recurrence.

- Younger Age - Women who are under 45 years of age are also at higher risk for recurrence after undergoing breast-conserving surgery.

If local recurrence occurs following breast-conserving surgery for DCIS, it is usually treated by completion (salvage) mastectomy. Recurrence after mastectomy, however, is very rare.

Breast Reconstruction for Ductal Carcinoma in Situ

Breast reconstruction is a surgical procedure to rebuild the breast and, if desired, the nipple and areola for women who have undergone a mastectomy. If mastectomy is the treatment of choice for ductal carcinoma in situ (DCIS), a skin-sparing approach, removing only the skin of the nipple-areola and the biopsy scar, facilitates breast reconstruction.

In general, there are two primary methods of breast reconstruction:

- Implant (tissue or skin expander) - During this procedure, a balloon expander is inserted under the skin and chest muscles and is periodically injected with a salt-water solution to fill the expander. The balloon expander is then removed and a permanent implant (saline or silicone) is implanted into the breast.

- Muscle Flap - During this procedure, a flap of muscle is transferred from another area of the body to the breast. A common type of muscle flap used for breast reconstruction is the TRAM flap which uses a flap of the lower abdominal wall fat to reconstruct the breast defect.

The Role of Complementary and Alternative Therapies in Cancer

Complementary and Alternative Medicine: Definition of Terms

The National Center for Complementary and Alternative Medicine (NCCAM) defines complementary and alternative medicine (CAM) as "a group of diverse medical and health care systems, practices, and products that are not presently considered to be a part of conventional medicine". The term **complementary medicine** refers to the use of CAM therapies in addition to or in conjunction with conventional mainstream treatments in an "integrative" approach to treatment. The term **alternative medicine**, on the other hand, refers to the use of CAM therapies as a substitute for or in place of conventional mainstream treatments.

Although the terms "complementary" and "alternative" are often used interchangeably by many people when referring to CAM therapies, health care professionals usually make a clear distinction between these two terms. In general, conventional physicians will keep an open mind and tend to support the use of "complementary" therapies in conjunction with standard mainstream treatments while they may resist suggestions for using "alternative" therapies as a substitute for conventional treatments. In fact, many cancer centers in the United States have incorporated select complementary therapies along with standard cancer treatments (e.g., chemotherapy, radiation therapy, surgery) in an emerging field of cancer care known as *integrative oncology*. It is important for patients and their families to keep in mind the very important distinction between the terms "complementary" and "alternative" when discussing the issue of CAM therapies with their health care provider in order to avoid confusion and misunderstandings and ensure effective patient-doctor communication.

The definition of CAM adapted by the NCCAM, which basically defines CAM as any treatment modality, philosophy, or product that falls outside the realm of conventional or standard medical care is well-suited for most Western countries where conventional, modern medicine is the prevailing or predominant health system adapted by the people who live in that culture. For example, conventional or standard treatments for cancer in most modern Western countries include chemotherapy, radiation therapy, biological therapy, and surgery. Other treatment modalities such as acupuncture, hypnotherapy, or the use of shark cartilage would be considered as being outside the realm of conventional medicine and falling under the general umbrella of CAM. The definition of CAM adapted by the NCCAM, however, is more problematic in countries or cultures where a particular form of CAM, such as Traditional Chinese medicine in China or Ayurvedic medicine in India, represent major health care systems that are recognized, accepted, and utilized by the general population of those countries or cultures.

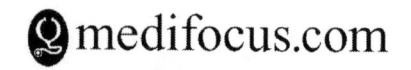

Care Versus Cure

In discussing the role of CAM therapies for the management of cancer, it is important to differentiate between CAM therapies that purport to "cure" cancer as opposed to those therapies that are used in palliative cancer care to provide relief from cancer-related symptoms and improve the patient's quality of life. Unlike some conventional cancer treatments that have been demonstrated to cure patients with certain types of cancers, currently there is a lack of sufficient scientific evidence to support the conclusion that any specific type of CAM modality can cure cancer. Patients who fail to draw a distinction between the "care versus cure" aspects of CAM therapies may delay seeking or may completely abandon potentially curative mainstream cancer treatments in hope that a particular CAM therapy may be a "magic bullet" for curing their cancer. On the other hand, complementary therapies have become an important aspect of palliative cancer care by helping cancer patients better cope with cancer-related symptoms and side-effects and, thereby, improving quality of life. In fact, many cancer centers in the United States and other Western countries have integrated complementary therapies into their mainstream treatment strategies for palliative cancer care in an emerging field of cancer practice known as *integrative oncology*.

Complementary Therapies for Cancer-Related Symptoms

Conventional cancer treatments such as chemotherapy, radiation therapy, and surgery are often associated with severe side-effects that can significantly impact the patient's quality of life and interfere with routine activities of daily living. In general, side-effects of conventional chemotherapy may include nausea/vomiting, fatigue, anxiety, depression, pain, sleep disturbances, loss of appetite, dry mouth, gastrointestinal disturbances, and peripheral neuropathy. Conventional treatments may not always be completely effective in relieving cancer-related symptoms and, in some cases, the treatments themselves may cause additional side-effects. Complementary therapies, when used in conjunction with conventional mainstream treatments can help patients better cope with cancer-related symptoms and side-effects and also improve physical and emotional well-being and overall quality of life.

Psychological Stress

The diagnosis of cancer is a life-altering event that may evoke feelings of anxiety, fear, depression, hopelessness, and severe psychological stress in many patients. Studies have shown that about 25% of cancer patients suffer from depression. Conventional treatments for anxiety, stress, and depression may involve the administration of anti-anxiety medications or antidepressants which may cause undesirable side-effects in some patients. Studies have shown that a variety of CAM therapies are useful for controlling anxiety and other mood disturbances when used in conjunction with conventional treatments. These include:

- Mind-body interventions - relaxation techniques, guided-imagery, meditation, hypnosis
- Acupuncture
- Massage therapy
- Music therapy

In general, patients with severe mood disturbances (e.g., panic attacks; suicide ideation) require immediate psychological evaluation and treatment to stabilize their acute condition before CAM therapies may be considered. For most patients with mild to moderate anxiety and mood disturbances, CAM therapies are a useful adjunct to conventional treatments for managing psychological distress. Techniques such as mind-body interventions, acupuncture, and music therapy are generally safe when performed by qualified, experienced practitioners and can help cancer patients better cope with feelings of anxiety, fear, hopelessness, and depression. Although some herbs and dietary supplements (e.g., Kava Kava; St. John's Wort; Passionflower) have been reported to relieve anxiety and mood disturbances, some experts have discouraged the use of these products in cancer patients because they may interfere with drugs used to treat cancer (chemotherapeutic agents) and/or other medications that patients may be taking. Patients should discuss the risks and benefits of using any herbal medications/dietary supplements with their oncologist before taking any of these products.

Cancer-Related Pain

Pain is a common symptom that can affect many cancer patients. Most often, the source of the pain is the tumor itself. Cancer-related pain may be caused by spread of the tumor to other tissues and organs or may result from compression of the tumor on a nerve or the spinal cord. In general, *acute* cancer-related pain is most responsive to conventional mainstream treatments which may involve medications (e.g., narcotic analgesics; steroids) or, in severe cases, (e.g., tumor causing spinal cord compression; tumor associated with abdominal obstruction), emergent surgery may be required to relieve the acute pain.

As a general rule, CAM therapies are usually not considered as a viable treatment option for the management of acute cancer-related pain. Once the acute pain has been brought under control by conventional treatment modalities, CAM therapies may be considered in the management of *chronic* cancer-related pain. A potential benefit of using CAM therapies in conjunction with conventional treatments for the management of chronic cancer-related pain is that they may reduce the dosage of conventional pain medications that may be required to achieve chronic pain control and, therefore, also potentially reduce the side-effects that may be associated with conventional pain medications.

A variety of CAM therapies, when used in conjunction with conventional treatments, may be beneficial for the management of cancer-related pain, including:

- Meditation
- Guided imagery
- Hypnosis
- Relaxation techniques
- Massage therapy
- Reflexology
- Acupuncture
- Yoga
- Aromatherapy

Some procedures that may be used for the diagnosis and treatment of some types of cancers may also be associated with pain. Examples include:

- Tissue biopsy - a piece of tissue is removed from the tumor and is examined under a microscope to determine if it is malignant or benign.
- Placement of a central line catheter that is used to administer chemotherapeutic agents and/or other medications
- Bone marrow aspiration
- Lumbar puncture (spinal tap)

A variety of CAM therapies, particularly mind-body techniques, have been found to be beneficial for controlling pain associated with cancer-related procedures (both diagnostic and therapeutic), especially in children with cancer, although they appear to be useful in adults as well.

Some cancer patients who undergo surgery to remove a tumor develop persistent neuropathic pain due to injury of nerves during the surgical procedure. In general, severe neuropathic pain may be difficult to control with conventional pain management treatment modalities. There is some evidence that acupuncture, when used in conjunction with conventional pain management strategies, may be effective for the management of persistent neuropathic pain that may develop in some patients after cancer surgery.

Nausea and Vomiting

Nausea and vomiting are relatively common side-effects in patients undergoing cancer chemotherapy. When used in conjunction with standard treatments, CAM therapies may offer patients additional relief from chemotherapy-induced nausea and vomiting. A 1998 National Institutes of Health (NIH) Consensus Conference concluded that there is clear evidence supporting the efficacy of acupuncture for controlling nausea and vomiting associated with cancer chemotherapy. Other CAM therapies that may help cancer patients better cope with chemotherapy-induced nausea and vomiting include:

- Acupressure
- Aromatherapy
- Hypnosis
- Guided imagery
- Music therapy
- Massage therapy

Other Cancer-Related Symptoms

There is a limited amount of evidence which suggests that CAM therapies may be useful for helping patients to better cope with a variety of other common cancer-related symptoms including:

- Fatigue - Studies have shown that acupuncture may be useful for reducing cancer-related fatigue in some patients.

- Dry Mouth (*xerostomia*) - Several studies suggest that acupuncture may be useful in the management of dry mouth that occurs in some patients undergoing radiation therapy to the head and neck.

- Hot Flashes - Some women with breast cancer who are treated with a drug called *tamoxifen* may experience hot flashes that can be very uncomfortable. Acupuncture may relieve menopause-related symptoms, including hot flashes, in women taking tamoxifen.

- Lymphedema - A specific type of massage therapy known as *manual lymphatic drainage* (MLD) is beneficial for the treatment of breast cancer related lymphedema and can also improve overall quality of life.

- Insomnia - A variety of mind-body therapies (e.g., relaxation techniques; meditation; biofeedback) may help to improve the quality of sleep of cancer patients who experience insomnia.

Dietary Modification and Supplementation

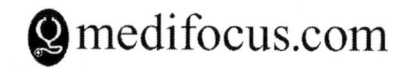

Evidence from epidemiological studies strongly supports a relationship between dietary factors and the risk for developing certain types of cancers. In general, a diet that is rich in certain food constituents (e.g., fruits, vegetable, fiber) appears to be protective against the development of cancer. In contrast, excessive consumption of other dietary substances (e.g., animal fats, alcohol) appears to increase the risk of certain types of cancers. Some vitamins that possess antioxidant properties (e.g., vitamins A, C, and E) may protect against certain types of cancers by protecting the body's cells from damage by certain compounds known as *free radicals*.

The role of dietary modification and antioxidant vitamin supplementation in slowing the progression of cancer continues to be an area of ongoing research. Currently, there are no conclusive studies which prove that any type of dietary modification or antioxidant vitamin supplementation can alter the progression of the disease in cancer patients.

Cancer patients who are considering dietary modification and/or antioxidant vitamin supplementation need to be aware of certain risks that may be associated with these regimens:

- Unintentional weight loss is a relatively common side-effect of cancer treatment, particularly among patients who are undergoing chemotherapy and/or radiation therapy. Excessive reduction of certain dietary components, such as dietary fat intake, may increase the risk of malnutrition in cancer patients. It is, therefore, important for patients to discuss the potential risks and benefits of any dietary modification with their oncologist before making a decision to modify their dietary intake.

- Some radical dietary regimens, such as *macrobiotic diets* (that are primarily vegetarian) may potentially promote the progression of disease in women with estrogen-receptor positive breast cancer or endometrial cancer due to their high content of isoflavonoid phytoestrogens. The same concern applies to diets that promote soy supplementation as a means of slowing the progression of cancer. Soy products contain high amounts of isoflavonoid phytoestrogens and should be avoided by women with estrogen-receptor positive tumors.

- High doses of certain antioxidant vitamin supplements (vitamins C and E) may increase the risk of bleeding complications in patients who have low levels of platelets in the bloodstream (thrombocytopenia) or patients who are taking anticoagulant medications. High doses of vitamin A can cause a condition called *Hypervitaminosis A* (Vitamin A toxicity) that can cause symptoms such as nausea, vomiting, headaches, blurry vision, and impaired consciousness.

Nutrition During Cancer Treatment and Recovery

In the past, many patients with cancer were diagnosed in the advanced stages of the disease when they may have already experienced the weight loss and cachexia (weakness and wasting of the body) that is common among patients with late-stage cancer. Since the advent of more effective cancer-screening techniques, however, more people are being diagnosed with early-stage cancer and many of these patients are already overweight or obese. In addition, all of the major cancer treatment modalities such as chemotherapy, radiation therapy, and surgery can significantly affect nutritional needs and alter eating habits. For these reasons, the American Cancer Society recommends that cancer patients undergoing active cancer treatment as well as cancer survivors who have completed therapy should ask their health care provider for a referral to see a registered dietician (RD), preferably one who is also a certified specialist in oncology (CSO). Nutritional assessment should begin as soon as possible after a cancer diagnosis and should focus on both the patient's current nutritional status as well as on anticipated nutritional deficiencies that may arise.

During cancer treatment, the goals of nutritional care should be to:

- Prevent or resolve nutritional deficiencies
- Achieve or maintain a healthy weight
- Preserve lean body mass
- Maximize quality of life

Individualized nutritional counseling during cancer treatment can:

- Reduce treatment-related side-effects
- Improve dietary intake
- Improve quality of life

Individualized nutritional counseling is of particular benefit under certain circumstances such as:

- For patients experiencing anorexia or early satiety who are at risk of becoming underweight, consuming smaller, more frequent meals with minimal liquids can help to increase food intake. Liquids, however, should be consumed in between meals to prevent dehydration.

- For cancer patients whose nutritional needs cannot be met through foods alone, fortified nutrient-dense foods or beverages can improve nutrition.

- Cancer patients who are at risk of becoming malnourished, other means of nutritional support may be needed such as appetite stimulants, a feeding tube, or intravenous parenteral nutrition.

Herbal Products

Currently there is a lack of sufficient scientific evidence to recommend the use of herbal products or supplements for the treatment of cancer. The safety of herbal formulations and products is also a major factor that should be taken into consideration by consumers. The National Center for Complementary and Alternative Medicine (NCCAM) urges consumers to be aware of several important safety issues pertaining to herbal products and supplements, including:

- Do not assume that just because many of these products are labeled as "natural", that they are necessarily safe and, therefore, cannot cause potentially serious adverse reactions. If you have any concerns about the possible side-effects of a particular herbal product or supplement, ask a pharmacist or your doctor about possible side-effects or interactions with other medications that you may be taking.

- Women who are pregnant or who are nursing should be especially cautious about using herbal products and supplements since the safety of many of these products has not established for use during pregnancy or lactation.

- Find out as much information as you can about a particular herbal product you are considering before taking it. If you have concerns or questions about a product, speak to a health care professional and get their advice. Moreover, you should always only use these products under the guidance of a health care professional.

- Some herbal products and supplements may interact with other medications that you may be taking and may cause adverse side-effects. Some herbal products may interfere with the action of certain chemotherapeutic agents that are used in the treatment of cancer. It is, therefore, important to notify your doctor about any herbal products you may be using or are considering using in order to prevent or reduce the possibility of adverse herb/drug interactions.

The use of vitamins, minerals, and other dietary supplements during cancer treatment is controversial. The American Cancer Society recommends that individuals should first assess whether they are nutrient deficient and limit use to those dietary supplements needed to treat a deficiency or promote another aspect of health. Cancer patients should also consider limiting dietary supplement use to therapeutic interventions for chronic conditions such as osteoporosis or macular degeneration, for which scientific evidence supports the likelihood of benefits.

The American Cancer Society also recommends that cancer survivors should strive to:

- Achieve and maintain a healthy weight.
- If overweight or obese, limit consumption of high-calorie foods and beverages and increase physical activity to promote weight loss.
- Achieve a dietary pattern that is high in fruits, vegetables, and whole grains.

Quality of Life Issues in Cancer

The diagnosis of any type of cancer is a frightening, life-altering event for both the patient and their family. The potential for a diminished quality of life for newly diagnosed cancer patients becomes an immediate, pressing concern when confronted with anxiety, fear, pain, the prospect of a long course of treatments that may cause significant side effects, and the possibility that the treatments may not work. It is critically important, however, for cancer patients and their families to address and learn to cope with the physical, emotional, and social issues that, if ignored and left to "fester", can rapidly lead to a significantly reduced quality of life.

Over the years, cancer specialists and other allied health-care professionals have come to realize that addressing a cancer patient's quality of life issues is an integral component of a comprehensive, overall cancer treatment strategy. From a practical perspective, that means developing an effective treatment plan that aims not only to control and/or to eradicate the patient's cancer with medical and/or surgical therapy but, at the same time, also takes into consideration critical issues of supportive care throughout the course of treatment and offers the patient the best chances of maintaining a reasonably high level quality of life. In fact, most cancer specialists now consider supportive care as an essential component of an overall, effective cancer treatment plan.

Factors Affecting Quality of Life in Cancer Patients

Cancer patients are confronted with a variety of physical, emotional, and social issues that, if left unchecked or ignored, can rapidly contribute to a diminished quality of life. In general, some of the more common problems encountered by cancer patients either as a result of the disease itself or as a side-effect of cancer treatments include:

- Sleep disorders
- Fatigue
- Diminished exercise capacity
- Unintentional weight loss
- Psychological stress
- Cancer-related pain

Sleep Disorders

Lack of adequate sleep due to anxiety, stress, pain, or treatment side-effects can lead to severe daytime fatigue that, in turn, can interfere with the ability to function and perform routine activities of daily living. Perhaps now, more than ever before, getting an adequate amount of sleep is critical to enable the body and mind to cope with the additional physical and emotional burdens resulting from cancer and its treatment. If sleep disturbances begin to affect your functional ability and diminish your quality of life, a variety of options are available to deal with the problem. These treatment options include learning new sleep habits (improved sleep hygiene practices); complementary therapies (e.g., relaxation techniques, biofeedback, meditation); and the use of prescription sleep medications. If lack of sleep is affecting your quality of life and interfering with your activities of daily living, talk with your doctor about developing an individualized treatment plan to help improve your quality of sleep.

Fatigue

Fatigue is perhaps the most common and potentially debilitating symptom experienced by cancer patients that can have a significant negative impact on routine activities of daily living and diminish quality of life. Fatigue may be attributed to a variety of causes including side-effects of cancer treatments (e.g., chemotherapy, radiation therapy), anemia, sleep deprivation resulting from insomnia, chronic pain, inadequate nutrition, and lack of physical exercise. In many cases, a combination of factors contributes to fatigue, exhaustion, and a general lack of energy. It is important to notify your cancer specialist or primary health care provider if you begin to experience bouts of fatigue lasting a few days or longer.

A variety of strategies are available to overcome the problem of fatigue in cancer patients. Fatigue related to anemia (low numbers of red blood cells) can be treated with blood transfusions and drugs, such as *erythropoietin* (e.g., Procrit) that promote the production of red blood cells. Fatigue not related to anemia may be managed with lifestyle modifications such as proper nutrition, regular exercise, and improved sleep hygiene practices.

Exercise

In the past, cancer patients were usually advised to "relax", "take it easy" and "don't overdo it". More recently, however, doctors are beginning to realize the potential benefits of physical exercise for cancer patients undergoing treatment as well as for cancer survivors. In general, the potential benefits of physical activity for patients suffering from chronic diseases include enhanced physical and mental function and improved quality of life. For cancer patients, the potential benefits of exercise also include decreased fatigue, improved appetite, better toleration of side effects of chemotherapy and radiation therapy and improved quality of life.

Studies have shown that physical activity after a cancer diagnosis is associated with a reduced risk of cancer recurrence and improved survival rates for several types of cancers including breast, prostate, colorectal, and ovarian cancer. Despite the many benefits of exercise, the American Cancer Society notes that the following precautions may be advisable for some cancer survivors:

- Survivors with severe anemia should delay exercise until the anemia is improved.

- Survivors with low white blood cell counts should avoid using public gyms and public pools until their white blood cell counts have returned to safe levels in order to prevent infections. Survivors who have undergone a bone marrow transplant should avoid these exposures for one year after transplantation.

- Survivors undergoing radiation therapy should avoid exposure to chlorine from swimming pools or other sources.

- Survivors with indwelling catheters or feeding tubes should avoid pool, lake, or ocean water to prevent microbial contamination and infection.

The American Cancer Society's recommendations for physical activity for cancer survivors includes:

- Engage in regular physical activity.
- Avoid inactivity and return to normal daily activity as soon as possible after diagnosis.
- Aim to exercise at least 150 minutes per week.
- Include strength-training exercises at least 2 days per week.

It is important, however, to speak to your cancer specialist about the types of exercises that may be appropriate at various stages of your cancer treatment and the types of physical activities that you should avoid.

Unintentional Weight Loss

One of the most common symptoms experienced by cancer patients is *unintentional weight loss* which can lead to malnutrition, increased susceptibility to infections, reduced quality of life, and shorter survival time. The underlying causes of unintentional weight loss in cancer patients may be attributed to a variety of factors including loss of appetite associated with chemotherapy and/or radiation therapy and psychological disturbances such as depression which has been found to affect up to 25% of cancer patients.

From a metabolic perspective, unintentional weight loss may be understood by the increased energy (calories) required by cancer cells to grow and spread as well as the increased energy requirements of the body to mount an effective response to fight the cancer. A net loss in weight occurs when the body uses more calories from stored energy reserves than is available from calories ingested from nutrients in the diet. Metabolic changes in cancer can also cause a condition called *cachexia* - a generalized wasting condition involving the loss of muscle mass and fat. Cachexia may develop even in people with good nutritional intake due to the failure of the body to absorb nutrients. Symptoms of cachexia, which affects about 50% of all cancer patients, include loss of appetite, weight loss, wasting of muscle mass, generalized fatigue, and significantly reduced capacity to perform routine activities of daily living.

The management of weight loss in cancer patients usually involves nutritional counseling to ensure an adequate intake of calories. Nutritional counseling can also help cancer patients develop new eating habits to prevent further weight loss including eating foods that are rich in calories or protein; eating smaller meals more frequently throughout the course of the day; "snacking" between meals; and drinking high-calorie liquid nutritional supplements (e.g., Boost, Ensure, Sustacal). In some cases, medications such as megestrol acetate (Megace) or dexamethasone (Decadron) may be prescribed to stimulate the appetite.

Your cancer specialist, working together with a nutritionist and a dietician, can help you develop and maintain a well-balanced diet to ensure that your body receives an adequate level of nutrition not only during the course of your cancer treatments but also during the recovery phase.

Psychological Stress

The diagnosis of cancer is a life-altering event that may evoke feelings of anxiety, fear, depression, hopelessness, and severe psychological stress in many patients. Studies have shown that about 25% of cancer patients suffer from depression. Conventional treatments for anxiety, stress, and depression may involve the administration of prescription anti-anxiety medications or antidepressants which may cause undesirable side-effects in some patients. Specific types of *psychotherapy* or "talk therapy" can also help relieve depression in cancer patients.

Studies have shown that a variety of complementary and alternative medicine (CAM) therapies are useful for controlling anxiety and other mood disturbances when used in conjunction with conventional treatments. These include:

- Mind-body interventions - relaxation techniques, guided-imagery, meditation, hypnosis
- Acupuncture
- Massage therapy
- Music therapy

In general, patients with severe mood disturbances (e.g., panic attacks; suicide ideation) require immediate psychological evaluation and treatment to stabilize their acute condition before CAM therapies may be considered. For most patients with mild to moderate anxiety and mood disturbances, CAM therapies are a useful adjunct to conventional treatments for managing psychological distress. Techniques such as mind-body interventions, acupuncture, and music therapy are generally safe when performed by qualified, experienced practitioners and can help cancer patients better cope with feelings of anxiety, fear, hopelessness, and depression. Although some herbs and dietary supplements (e.g., Kava Kava; St. John's Wort; Passionflower) have been reported to relieve anxiety and mood disturbances, some experts have discouraged the use of these products in cancer patients because they may interfere with drugs used to treat cancer (chemotherapeutic agents) and/or other medications that patients may be taking. Patients should discuss the risks and benefits of using any herbal medications/dietary supplements with their oncologist before taking any of these products, particularly if they are undergoing chemotherapy, radiation therapy, or surgery.

Cancer-Related Pain

Pain is a relatively common symptom that is experienced by many cancer patients. In recent years, increased awareness about this problem has led to important advances in the management of patients with cancer-related pain. In fact, today most major cancer centers in the United States have established pain management clinics, usually located within the Anesthesiology department of a hospital, that specialize in helping patients to better control their cancer-related pain.

Most often, the source of cancer-related pain is the tumor itself. This can occur when a tumor spreads and invades other tissues or organs of the body; when a tumor compresses a nearby nerve or the spinal cord; or when a tumor causes intestinal obstruction. Cancer-related pain may also be caused by some procedures that are used for the diagnosis and treatment of cancer. Examples include tissue biopsy; placement of a central line catheter; bone marrow aspiration; and spinal tap.

Irrespective of the source of your cancer pain, it is important to notify your oncologist or primary care doctor about any pain or discomfort that you may be experiencing so that appropriate measures can be taken to eliminate or better control the pain. In developing an individualized pain control strategy, your doctor will want to learn as much as possible about the pain you are experiencing, including:

- When did the pain start?
- How long does the pain last (acute or chronic)?
- Is the pain minor, moderate, or severe?
- Is the pain localized to a particular area of the body?
- Are there any specific activities or events that either "trigger" the pain or help to alleviate the pain?
- To what extent does the pain interfere with your quality of life and activities of daily living?

- Are you currently taking any pain medications?

Drug Therapy for Cancer-Related Pain

A wide range of pain medications is available for helping patients better cope with cancer-related pain. Your doctor will determine the specific type of medication that is most suitable for you based on the information you provide including the severity of the pain (e.g., mild, moderate, or severe) and the duration of the pain. You can help your doctor in selecting the most appropriate pain medication for your specific type of cancer pain by providing him/her with as much information as possible about the nature and characteristics of the pain. Be sure to also notify your doctor if:

- You are allergic to any medications
- You have previously experienced any serious side-effects from pain medications (e.g., gastrointestinal bleeding)
- You have a current or past history of stomach ulcers
- You are taking any other pain medications including herbal products or medications.

In general, the following pain medication treatment options are available in the management of cancer-related pain based upon the severity of the pain:

- Non-Steroidal Anti-Inflammatory Drugs - Mild cancer-related pain can usually be managed with a variety of pain medications that belong to the general family of drugs known as *non-steroidal anti-inflammatory drugs* (NSAIDs). Examples of NSAIDs that are available "over-the-counter" include:

  - aspirin (e.g., Bayer)
  - acetaminophen (e.g., Tylenol)
  - ibuprofen (e.g., Motrin)
  - naproxen (e.g., Aleve)

Some NSAIDs used for the treatment of pain, including cancer-related pain, are available by prescription only. Examples include diclofenac (e.g., Voltaren); indomethacin (Indocin); ketoprofen (e.g., Orudis); and Cox-2 inhibitors (e.g., Celebrex), among others.

- Narcotic (Opioid) Analgesics - If you are experiencing mild to moderate cancer-related pain, your doctor may prescribe a medication that belongs to a family of drugs known as *narcotic analgesics*. Examples include:

  - codeine
  - morphine
  - buprenorphine (e.g., Subutex; Suboxone)

- fentanyl (e.g., Duragesic)
- oxycodone (e.g., OxyNorm; OxyContin)
- hydrocodone (e.g., Vicodin; Lortab)
- hydromorphone (e.g., Dilaudid)

In some cases, combination pain medication tablets containing an NSAID plus a narcotic analgesic may be prescribed for the management of mild to moderate cancer-related pain. Examples of combination pain medication tablets include Percodan (aspirin plus oxycodone); Percocet (acetaminophen plus oxycodone); Co-codamol (acetaminophen plus codeine); and Co-codaprin (aspirin plus codeine).

As a general "rule of thumb", cancer patients with mild to moderate pain are usually started on "weaker" opioid-based medications (e.g., codeine) and, if necessary, are switched to stronger opioid medications (e.g., fentanyl, oxycodone, morphine).

Common side-effects of narcotic analgesics include constipation, lethargy, drowsiness, nausea/vomiting, and sleepiness. In addition, a major concern with the use of narcotic analgesics is the possibility of addiction to the medications. Be sure you notify your doctor if you have a current or past history of drug and/or alcohol abuse before taking narcotic analgesics. Also speak with your doctor about strategies that can be used to manage the side-effects of narcotic analgesics. For example, constipation may be managed by taking a stool softener (e.g., Colace; Senokot). If you experience drowsiness or sleepiness when you take your pain medication, you should avoid any activities that may pose a danger to yourself or others (e.g., driving a car; mowing the lawn).

- Adjuvant Pain Medications - Some drugs that are primary used to treat conditions other than pain also possess analgesic (pain-relieving) properties. These drugs are known as *adjuvant pain medications* and are sometimes prescribed, alone or in combination with other medications, for the management of cancer-related pain. Examples include:

  - anticonvulsants - This class of drugs is used primarily to treat seizures. Examples of anticonvulsants that may also be used to treat cancer pain include: gabapentin (e.g.,Neurontin); carbamazepine (e.g., Tegretol); phenytoin (e.g., Dilantin); and topiramate (e.g., Topamax)

  - antidepressants - This class of drugs is used primarily to treat depression. Examples of antidepressants that may be also be used to treat cancer pain include: amitriptylene (e.g., Elavil); desipramine (e.g., Norpramin); doxepin (e.g., Sinequon); and impipramine (e.g., Tofranil).

- bisphosphonates - This class of drugs is used primarily for the treatment of osteoporosis. Studies have also demonstrated that bisphosphonates may relieve bone pain in cancer patients. Examples include: alendronate (e.g., Fosamax); pamidronate (Aredia); and etidronate (e.g., Didronel).

- corticosteroids - This class of drugs is used primarily to treat inflammatory conditions such as rheumatoid arthritis, osteoarthritis, and ankylosing spondylitis. By reducing inflammation, corticosteroids also reduce pain. A common type of corticosteroid drug used for the management of cancer pain is dexamethasone (e.g., Dexmethsone).

- Breakthrough Cancer Pain - Despite the regular use of pain medications on a fixed schedule, many cancer patients (estimates range from 50% to 65%) experience a type of pain known as *breakthrough cancer pain*. This type of pain is characterized by a sudden onset, may last from minutes to hours, and is usually severe in nature. Breakthrough cancer pain occurs most often in patients who are experiencing persistent or chronic cancer pain who notice a sudden, periodic "flare-up" of severe pain even though they are taking pain medication on a regular schedule.

Breakthrough cancer pain is most often treated with opioid medications that act quickly, such as immediate release morphine tablets or capsules, but are rapidly eliminated from the body so that they cause less side-effects. The U.S. Food and Drug Administration (FDA) has also approved a drug called ACTIQ (Oral Transmucosal Fentanyl Citrate) in the form of a lozenge on a stick that dissolves slowly in the mouth for the treatment of breakthrough cancer pain. Be sure to notify your doctor if you think you may be experiencing breakthrough pain that is not controlled with your regular fixed-schedule pain medications so that he/she may determine the best course of treatment to alleviate your pain.

For more information about cancer-related pain and the treatment options, please click on the following link: http://www.cancer-pain.org

The Role of Complementary and Alternative Medicine Therapies in Cancer-Related Pain

As a general rule, complementary and alternative medicine (CAM) therapies are usually not considered as a viable treatment option for the management of acute cancer-related pain. Acute cancer-related pain usually responds best to conventional drug therapy (e.g., NSAIDs; narcotic analgesics; adjuvant pain medications). Surgery may also be necessary for the treatment of some types of acute cancer pain such as when a tumor compresses a nearby nerve or the spinal cord or if the tumor is causing abdominal or intestinal obstruction. Once the acute pain has been brought under control by conventional treatment modalities, CAM therapies may be considered in the management of *chronic* (persistent) cancer-related pain. A potential benefit of using CAM therapies in conjunction with conventional treatments for the management of chronic cancer-related pain is that they may reduce the dosage of conventional pain medications that may be required to achieve chronic pain control and, therefore, also potentially reduce the side-effects that may be associated with conventional pain medications.

A variety of CAM therapies, when used in conjunction with conventional treatments, may be beneficial for the management of chronic cancer-related pain, including:

- Meditation
- Guided imagery
- Hypnosis
- Relaxation techniques
- Massage therapy
- Reflexology
- Acupuncture
- Yoga
- Aromatherapy

Where Can You Find Supportive Care?

Fortunately, supportive care is available for cancer patients and their families from a multitude of resources. These include:

- Cancer Centers - the hospital or cancer center where you have chosen to receive your treatment is an excellent starting point in your search for supportive cancer care. Many major hospitals and comprehensive cancer centers provide access to a variety of resources for cancer patients including educational, psychological, and social services support.

- Your Cancer Physician - the primary cancer specialist who is in charge of your care and is responsible for your overall treatment is also an excellent resource of information and support. These cancer specialists are in the business of caring for cancer patients and usually have a wealth of knowledge about the physical, psychological, and social issues confronting patients who have been diagnosed with cancer. Depending upon your specific type of cancer, a variety of cancer specialists may be involved in your treatment including an:

    - oncologist
    - hematologist

- radiation oncologist
- surgical oncologist

- Oncology Nurses - if your treatment plan includes chemotherapy, you will be assigned a nurse oncologist who will administer your drugs and monitor side-effects or other problems that may occur during your chemotherapy sessions. Nurse oncologists are highly trained professionals who are a wonderful source of information and can provide educational materials, emotional support, and practical tips for dealing with adverse side-effects of chemotherapy such as nausea, fatigue, and pain.

- Your Primary Care Physician - it is likely that a visit to your primary care physician led to the discovery and diagnosis of your cancer and that your primary care physician referred you to a cancer specialist for treatment. Your primary care physician will usually work closely with your cancer specialist in following your progress both during as well as after treatment has been completed. It is important to be open and frank with your primary care physician and talk to him/her about any physical or emotional problems that you may experience so that they can help you get over these difficult periods.

- Nurse Practitioners - Nurse practitioners are registered nurses (RNs) who have completed additional courses and training. They can work with or without the supervision of a physician. Their scope of work includes both diagnosis and treatment of diseases and, in many states, they can also write prescriptions.

- Physician's Assistants - A physician's assistant is a licensed health care professional who provides care under the supervision of a physician. Physician's assistants provide a broad range of diagnostic and therapeutic services including ordering and interpreting laboratory tests, diagnosing and treating diseases and conditions, conducting physical examinations, and assisting in surgery.

- Nutritionists/Dieticians - consultation with a nutritional expert can help ensure that you maintain an adequate level of nutrition throughout your cancer treatment and that your body has sufficient energy to withstand the rigorous cancer treatments which may carry significant side-effects. Well-nourished cancer patients also have more energy and are less prone to experience severe fatigue and exhaustion.

- Social Workers - a social worker who is experienced in working with cancer patients (oncology social workers) can provide valuable assistance in dealing with a variety of social and emotional issues including:

    - teaching patients and families to navigate the complexities of the health-care

system
- helping with financial and health insurance issues
- assisting family members in adjusting to new roles and responsibilities
- arranging home health care for patients requiring home-based treatments
- providing access to local, state, and government agencies that provide social and health services
- helping cancer patients deal with employees and return to work issues

- Mental Health Professionals - A psychiatrist or psychologist with expertise in diagnosing and treating psychological and emotional disturbances in cancer patients (e.g., anxiety, fear, depression, self-image issues) is an integral member of the comprehensive cancer team who can help patients better cope and adjust to living with cancer.

- Clergy - a trusted member of the clergy can provide spiritual guidance, reassurance, and hope to cancer patients and their families.

- Sex Therapists - a sex therapist can help cancer patients who experience a reduced libido or other sexual problems that may develop as a consequence of the cancer itself or treatment related side-effects.

- Family and Friends - family, friends, and long-term acquaintances who know you best are one of your most important support networks and can provide emotional support, guidance, and encouragement both during and long after you've completed your course of cancer therapy. Now, more than ever, you need to open-up to your family and friends and share your feelings, fears, and emotions with them. They will appreciate your willingness to trust and confide in them and you will benefit from their reassurance, encouragement, positive attitude, and continuous love.

- Organizations and Support Groups - a broad range of organizations and support groups that specialize in helping cancer patients and their families represent a valuable source of support, networking, access to services, and for obtaining important educational cancer materials. Some of these major organizations may be located in your city and some cancer support groups may even have branches in your neighborhood. Joining a cancer support group may be one of the most important steps you take to help yourself on the road to recovery. Networking and "connecting" with other cancer patients and cancer survivors who understand and share your fears and concerns can be an important source of consolation, comfort, and peace of mind knowing that you are not alone in this battle. Other cancer patients have been down this road before and learning about their personal experiences and coping strategies can help you work your way through this difficult period in your life.

New Developments in Ductal Carcinoma in Situ

- Research is ongoing to better define the role of adjuvant hormonal therapy in the management of women with ductal carcinoma in Situ (DCIS).

- Research is ongoing to better define the role of radiation therapy in the management of women with DCIS.

- Research is ongoing to more accurately identify women with DCIS who are at high risk for recurrence of breast cancer (invasive or in situ).

- Newer imaging techniques are being investigated to improve the accuracy of early breast cancer screening and detection.

- The role of oral contraceptives as a risk factor for DCIS is being investigated.

- The use of biological markers that can potentially more accurately predict the risk of recurrence in patients with DCIS following surgery is being investigated.

- The risk of recurrence following treatment of DCIS with skin-sparing mastectomy and immediate breast reconstruction is under investigation.

- The potential role of newer selective estrogen receptor modulators (SERMs) as adjuvant therapy in women with estrogen-receptor positive DCIS is being investigated.

- The role of cyclo-oxygenase 2 (COX-2) inhibitors in the treatment of DCIS is under investigation.

- *Mammary ductoscopy*, a new imaging technique that allows doctors to better visualize the ductal system of the breasts, is emerging as a potentially important tool in guiding breast-conserving surgery for DCIS.

- Information regarding ongoing clinical studies in your area can be obtained at the Clinical Trials Listing Service at http://www.centerwatch.com

Questions to Ask Your Health Care Provider About Ductal Carcinoma in Situ

- What is the nuclear-grade of my DCIS (high, low, or intermediate)?
- What type of surgery do you recommend for my type of DCIS and why?
- What are the risks and complications of surgery for DCIS?
- Will I also require radiation therapy after surgery?
- Will I need adjuvant hormonal therapy with tamoxifen?
- What are the risks and benefits of tamoxifen therapy?
- What is the long-term prognosis for my type of DCIS?
- What is the likelihood that my DCIS will recur after treatment?
- What ongoing monitoring will be necessary to detect any recurrence?

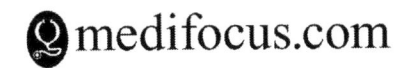

NOTES

Use this page for taking notes as you review your Guidebook

3 - Guide to the Medical Literature

Introduction

This section of your *MediFocus Guidebook* is a comprehensive bibliography of important recent medical literature published about the condition from authoritative, trustworthy medical journals. This is the same information that is used by physicians and researchers to keep up with the latest advances in clinical medicine and biomedical research. A broad spectrum of articles is included in each *MediFocus Guidebook* to provide information about standard treatments, treatment options, new developments, and advances in research.

To facilitate your review and analysis of this information, the articles in this *MediFocus Guidebook* are grouped in the following categories:

- Review Articles - 39 Articles
- General Interest Articles - 74 Articles
- Drug Therapy Articles - 2 Articles
- Surgical Therapy Articles - 28 Articles
- Clinical Trials Articles - 11 Articles
- Radiation Therapy Articles - 12 Articles

The following information is provided for each of the articles referenced in this section of your *MediFocus Guidebook*:

- Title of the article
- Name of the authors
- Institution where the study was done
- Journal reference (Volume, page numbers, year of publication)
- Link to Abstract (brief summary of the actual article)

Linking to Abstracts: Most of the medical journal articles referenced in this section of your *MediFocus Guidebook* include an abstract (brief summary of the actual article) that can be accessed online via the National Library of Medicine's PubMed® database. You can easily access the individual article abstracts online by entering the individual URL address for a particular article into your web browser, or by going to the following special URL:

http://www.medifocus.com/links/OC008/0814

Recent Literature: What Your Doctor Reads

Database: PubMed <January 2010 to August 2014>

Review Articles

1.

Ductal carcinoma in situ of the breast: can biomarkers improve current management?

Authors:	Bartlett JM; Nofech-Moses S; Rakovitch E
Institution:	Ontario Institute for Cancer Research, Toronto, ON, Canada;
Journal:	Clin Chem. 2014 Jan;60(1):60-7. doi: 10.1373/clinchem.2013.207183. Epub 2013 Nov 21.
Abstract Link:	http://www.medifocus.com/abstracts.php?gid=OC008&ID=24262106

2.

Breast conserving therapy for DCIS--does size matter?

Authors:	Kantor O; Winchester DJ
Institution:	University of Chicago, Pritzker School of Medicine, Chicago, Illinois.
Journal:	J Surg Oncol. 2014 Jul;110(1):75-81. doi: 10.1002/jso.23657. Epub 2014 May 27.
Abstract Link:	http://www.medifocus.com/abstracts.php?gid=OC008&ID=24861481

3.

Predictors of recurrence for ductal carcinoma in situ after breast-conserving surgery.

Authors:	Benson JR; Wishart GC
Institution:	Cambridge Breast Unit, Addenbrooke's Hospital, Cambridge, UK; Anglia Ruskin University, Cambridge, UK. john.benson@addenbrookes.nhs.uk
Journal:	Lancet Oncol. 2013 Aug;14(9):e348-57. doi: 10.1016/S1470-2045(13)70135-9.
Abstract Link:	http://www.medifocus.com/abstracts.php?gid=OC008&ID=23896274

Go to http://www.medifocus.com/links/OC008/0814 for direct online access to the above Abstract Links.

4.

Is DCIS breast cancer, and how do I treat it?

Authors:	Bijker N; Donker M; Wesseling J; den Heeten GJ; Rutgers EJ
Institution:	Department of Radiation Oncology, Academic Medical Center, P.O. Box 22700, 1100DE, Amsterdam, The Netherlands. n.bijker@amc.uva.nl
Journal:	Curr Treat Options Oncol. 2013 Mar;14(1):75-87. doi: 10.1007/s11864-012-0217-1.
Abstract Link:	http://www.medifocus.com/abstracts.php?gid=OC008&ID=23239193

5.

Ductal carcinoma in situ.

Author:	Bleicher RJ
Institution:	Department of Surgical Oncology, Fox Chase Cancer Center, 333 Cottman Avenue, Room C-308, Philadelphia, PA 19111, USA. richard.bleicher@fccc.edu
Journal:	Surg Clin North Am. 2013 Apr;93(2):393-410. doi: 10.1016/j.suc.2012.12.001. Epub 2013 Jan 29.
Abstract Link:	http://www.medifocus.com/abstracts.php?gid=OC008&ID=23464692

6.

Breast ductal carcinoma in situ presenting as recurrent non-puerperal mastitis: case report and literature review.

Authors:	Liong YV; Hong GS; Teo JG; Lim GH
Institution:	Breast Department, KK Women's and Children's Hospital, Singapore, Singapore.
Journal:	World J Surg Oncol. 2013 Aug 7;11(1):179. doi: 10.1186/1477-7819-11-179.
Abstract Link:	http://www.medifocus.com/abstracts.php?gid=OC008&ID=23924035

Go to http://www.medifocus.com/links/OC008/0814 for direct online access to the above Abstract Links.

7.

Ductal carcinoma in situ of the breast: current concepts and future directions.

Author:	Siziopikou KP
Institution:	Breast Pathology Service, Northwestern University Feinberg School of Medicine, Chicago, Illinois, USA. p-siziopikou@northwestern.edu
Journal:	Arch Pathol Lab Med. 2013 Apr;137(4):462-6. doi: 10.5858/arpa.2012-0078-RA.
Abstract Link:	http://www.medifocus.com/abstracts.php?gid=OC008&ID=23544935

8.

Radiation therapy in the management of breast cancer.

Authors:	Yang TJ; Ho AY
Institution:	Department of Radiation Oncology, Memorial Sloan-Kettering Cancer Center, 1275 York Avenue, New York, NY 10065, USA.
Journal:	Surg Clin North Am. 2013 Apr;93(2):455-71. doi: 10.1016/j.suc.2013.01.002.
Abstract Link:	http://www.medifocus.com/abstracts.php?gid=OC008&ID=23464696

9.

Management of elderly patients with breast cancer: updated recommendations of the International Society of Geriatric Oncology (SIOG) and European Society of Breast Cancer Specialists (EUSOMA).

Authors:	Biganzoli L; Wildiers H; Oakman C; Marotti L; Loibl S; Kunkler I; Reed M; Ciatto S; Voogd AC; Brain E; Cutuli B; Terret C; Gosney M; Aapro M; Audisio R
Institution:	Sandro Pitigliani Medical Oncology Unit, Istituto Toscano Tumori, Hospital of Prato, Prato, Italy. lbiganzoli@usl4.toscana.it
Journal:	Lancet Oncol. 2012 Apr;13(4):e148-60. Epub 2012 Mar 30.
Abstract Link:	http://www.medifocus.com/abstracts.php?gid=OC008&ID=22469125

Go to http://www.medifocus.com/links/OC008/0814 for direct online access to the above Abstract Links.

10.

Why the term 'low-grade ductal carcinoma in situ' should be changed to 'borderline breast disease': diagnostic and clinical implications.

Author:	Masood S
Institution:	Department of Pathology, University of Florida College of Medicine, Jacksonville, FL, USA. shahla.masood@jax.ufl.edu
Journal:	Womens Health (Lond Engl). 2012 Jan;8(1):57-62.
Abstract Link:	http://www.medifocus.com/abstracts.php?gid=OC008&ID=22171775

11.

Breast microcalcifications as type descriptors to stratify risk of malignancy: a systematic review and meta-analysis of 10665 cases with special focus on round/punctate microcalcifications.

Authors:	Rominger M; Wisgickl C; Timmesfeld N
Institution:	Klinik fur Strahlendiagnostik, Klinikum der Philipps-Univ. Marburg, Marburg, Germany. rominger@med.uni-marburg.de
Journal:	Rofo. 2012 Dec;184(12):1144-52. doi: 10.1055/s-0032-1313102. Epub 2012 Aug 24.
Abstract Link:	http://www.medifocus.com/abstracts.php?gid=OC008&ID=22923222

12.

Ductal carcinoma in situ (DCIS) of the breast: perspectives on biology and controversies in current management.

Authors:	Schmale I; Liu S; Rayhanabad J; Russell CA; Sener SF
Institution:	Division of Breast and Soft Tissue Surgery, Department of Surgery, Keck School of Medicine, University of Southern California, Los Angeles, California, USA.
Journal:	J Surg Oncol. 2012 Feb;105(2):212-20. doi: 10.1002/jso.22020. Epub 2011 Jul 12.
Abstract Link:	http://www.medifocus.com/abstracts.php?gid=OC008&ID=21751217

Go to http://www.medifocus.com/links/OC008/0814 for direct online access to the above Abstract Links.

13.

Postoperative tamoxifen for ductal carcinoma in situ.

Authors:	Staley H; McCallum I; Bruce J
Institution:	Northumbria Healthcare NHS Foundation Trust, North Tyneside General Hospital, North Shields, UK.
Journal:	Cochrane Database Syst Rev. 2012 Oct 17;10:CD007847. doi: 10.1002/14651858.CD007847.pub2.
Abstract Link:	http://www.medifocus.com/abstracts.php?gid=OC008&ID=23076938

14.

Network meta-analysis of margin threshold for women with ductal carcinoma in situ.

Authors:	Wang SY; Chu H; Shamliyan T; Jalal H; Kuntz KM; Kane RL; Virnig BA
Institution:	Division of Health Policy and Management, University of Minnesota School of Public Health, 420 Delaware St S.E., MMC 729, Minneapolis, MN 55455, USA. wang1018@umn.edu
Journal:	J Natl Cancer Inst. 2012 Apr 4;104(7):507-16. Epub 2012 Mar 22.
Abstract Link:	http://www.medifocus.com/abstracts.php?gid=OC008&ID=22440677

15.

The molecular pathology of breast cancer progression.

Authors:	Bombonati A; Sgroi DC
Institution:	Department of Pathology, Harvard Medical School, Molecular Pathology Research Unit, Massachusetts General Hospital, Boston, MA, USA.
Journal:	J Pathol. 2011 Jan;223(2):307-17. doi: 10.1002/path.2808. Epub 2010 Nov 16.
Abstract Link:	http://www.medifocus.com/abstracts.php?gid=OC008&ID=21125683

Go to http://www.medifocus.com/links/OC008/0814 for direct online access to the above Abstract Links.

16.

Ductal carcinoma in situ: detection, diagnosis, and characterization with magnetic resonance imaging.

Author:	Jansen SA
Institution:	Mouse Cancer Genetics Program, National Cancer Institute, Frederick, MD, USA. jansena@mail.nih.gov
Journal:	Semin Ultrasound CT MR. 2011 Aug;32(4):306-18. doi: 10.1053/j.sult.2011.02.007.
Abstract Link:	http://www.medifocus.com/abstracts.php?gid=OC008&ID=21782121

17.

Ductal carcinoma in-situ: an update for clinical practice.

Authors:	Patani N; Khaled Y; Al Reefy S; Mokbel K
Institution:	The London Breast Institute, The Princess Grace Hospital, London, UK.
Journal:	Surg Oncol. 2011 Mar;20(1):e23-31. Epub 2010 Nov 24.
Abstract Link:	http://www.medifocus.com/abstracts.php?gid=OC008&ID=21106367

18.

Ductal carcinoma in situ: terminology, classification, and natural history.

Author:	Allred DC
Institution:	Department of Pathology and Immunology, Washington University School of Medicine, 660 South Euclid Ave, Campus Box 8118, St Louis, MO 63110, USA. dcallred@path.wustl.edu
Journal:	J Natl Cancer Inst Monogr. 2010;2010(41):134-8.
Abstract Link:	http://www.medifocus.com/abstracts.php?gid=OC008&ID=20956817

Go to http://www.medifocus.com/links/OC008/0814 for direct online access to the above Abstract Links.

19.

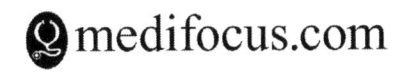

Risk of invasive breast cancer after lobular intra-epithelial neoplasia: review of the literature.

Authors:	Ansquer Y; Delaney S; Santulli P; Salomon L; Carbonne B; Salmon R
Institution:	Hopital St Antoine, Assistance Publique Hopitaux de Paris, Universite Pierre et Marie Curie, Paris VI, Service de Gynecologie Obstetrique, 184 rue du Faubourg St Antoine, 75012 Paris, Cedex 12, France. yan.ansquer@sat.aphp.fr
Journal:	Eur J Surg Oncol. 2010 Jul;36(7):604-9. Epub 2010 Jun 11.
Abstract Link:	http://www.medifocus.com/abstracts.php?gid=OC008&ID=20541352

20.

Local and systemic outcomes in DCIS based on tumor and patient characteristics: the radiation oncologist's perspective.

Authors:	Bijker N; van Tienhoven G
Institution:	Department of Radiotherapy, Academic Medical Centre, PO Box 22660, 1100 DD Amsterdam, the Netherlands. n.bijker@amc.uva.nl
Journal:	J Natl Cancer Inst Monogr. 2010;2010(41):178-80.
Abstract Link:	http://www.medifocus.com/abstracts.php?gid=OC008&ID=20956825

21.

Overview of the randomized trials of radiotherapy in ductal carcinoma in situ of the breast.

Authors:	Correa C; McGale P; Taylor C; Wang Y; Clarke M; Davies C; Peto R; Bijker N; Solin L; Darby S
Journal:	J Natl Cancer Inst Monogr. 2010;2010(41):162-77.
Abstract Link:	http://www.medifocus.com/abstracts.php?gid=OC008&ID=20956824

22.

Imaging for the diagnosis and management of ductal carcinoma in situ.

Author:	D'Orsi CJ
Institution:	Department of Radiology, Breast Imaging Center, Emory University Hospital, WCI Bldg, 1365-C Clifton Rd, Ste C1104, Atlanta, GA 30322, USA. carl_dorsi@emoryhealthcare.org
Journal:	J Natl Cancer Inst Monogr. 2010;2010(41):214-7.
Abstract Link:	http://www.medifocus.com/abstracts.php?gid=OC008&ID=20956833

23.

The impact of systemic therapy following ductal carcinoma in situ.

Authors:	Eng-Wong J; Costantino JP; Swain SM
Institution:	Department of Internal Medicine, Division of Oncology, Lombardi Cancer Center, Georgetown University, Washington, DC, USA.
Journal:	J Natl Cancer Inst Monogr. 2010;2010(41):200-3.
Abstract Link:	http://www.medifocus.com/abstracts.php?gid=OC008&ID=20956830

24.

Current perspectives of treatment of ductal carcinoma in situ.

Authors:	Estevez LG; Alvarez I; Segui MA; Munoz M; Margeli M; Miro C; Rubio C; Lluch A; Tusquets I
Institution:	Centro Integral Oncologico Clara Campal, Madrid, Spain. lauraestevez@hospitaldemadrid.com
Journal:	Cancer Treat Rev. 2010 Nov;36(7):507-17. Epub 2010 May 11.
Abstract Link:	http://www.medifocus.com/abstracts.php?gid=OC008&ID=20462701

Go to http://www.medifocus.com/links/OC008/0814 for direct online access to the above Abstract Links.

25.

Quality-of-life issues in patients with ductal carcinoma in situ.

Author:	Ganz PA
Institution:	Division of Cancer Prevention and Control Research, Jonsson Comprehensive Cancer Center, 650 Charles Young Dr South, Rm A2-125 CHS, Los Angeles, CA 90095-6900, USA. pganz@ucla.edu
Journal:	J Natl Cancer Inst Monogr. 2010;2010(41):218-22.
Abstract Link:	http://www.medifocus.com/abstracts.php?gid=OC008&ID=20956834

26.

The impact of surgery on ductal carcinoma in situ outcomes: the use of mastectomy.

Author:	Hwang ES
Institution:	Department of Surgery and Helen Diller Family Comprehensive Cancer Center, University of California, San Francisco, San Francisco, CA 94115, USA. shelley.hwang@ucsfmedctr.org
Journal:	J Natl Cancer Inst Monogr. 2010;2010(41):197-9.
Abstract Link:	http://www.medifocus.com/abstracts.php?gid=OC008&ID=20956829

27.

The impact of surgery, radiation, and systemic treatment on outcomes in patients with ductal carcinoma in situ.

Authors:	Kane RL; Virnig BA; Shamliyan T; Wang SY; Tuttle TM; Wilt TJ
Institution:	Division of Health Policy and Management, University of Minnesota School of Public Health, D351 Mayo (MMC 729), 420 Delaware St SE, Minneapolis, MN 55455, USA. kanex001@umn.edu
Journal:	J Natl Cancer Inst Monogr. 2010;2010(41):130-3.
Abstract Link:	http://www.medifocus.com/abstracts.php?gid=OC008&ID=20956816

Go to http://www.medifocus.com/links/OC008/0814 for direct online access to the above Abstract Links.

28.

Epidemiology of ductal carcinoma in situ.

Author:	Kerlikowske K
Institution:	General Internal Medicine Section, San Francisco Veterans Affairs Medical Center, University of California, San Francisco, 4150 Clement St, 111A1, San Francisco, CA 94121, USA. karla.kerlikowske@ucsf.edu
Journal:	J Natl Cancer Inst Monogr. 2010;2010(41):139-41.
Abstract Link:	http://www.medifocus.com/abstracts.php?gid=OC008&ID=20956818

29.

Magnetic resonance imaging in the evaluation of ductal carcinoma in situ.

Author:	Lehman CD
Institution:	Department of Radiology, University of Washington School of Medicine, Seattle Cancer Care Alliance, 825 Eastlake Ave E., G2-600, Seattle, WA 98109-1023, USA. lehman@u.washington.edu
Journal:	J Natl Cancer Inst Monogr. 2010;2010(41):150-1.
Abstract Link:	http://www.medifocus.com/abstracts.php?gid=OC008&ID=20956821

30.

Local control of ductal carcinoma in situ based on tumor and patient characteristics: the surgeon's perspective.

Author:	Newman LA
Institution:	Department of Surgery, Breast Care Center, University of Michigan Comprehensive Cancer Center, 1500 East Medical Center Dr, 3308 Cancer Center, Ann Arbor, MI 48109-0932, USA. lanewman@umich.edu
Journal:	J Natl Cancer Inst Monogr. 2010;2010(41):152-7.
Abstract Link:	http://www.medifocus.com/abstracts.php?gid=OC008&ID=20956822

Go to http://www.medifocus.com/links/OC008/0814 for direct online access to the above Abstract Links.

31.

Mode of detection and secular time for ductal carcinoma in situ.

Author:	Pisano ED
Institution:	Department of Radiology, Medical University of South Carolina College of Medicine, 96 Jonathan Lucas Street, Suite 601, MSC 617. Charleston, SC 29425, USA. pisanoe@musc.edu
Journal:	J Natl Cancer Inst Monogr. 2010;2010(41):142-4.
Abstract Link:	http://www.medifocus.com/abstracts.php?gid=OC008&ID=20956819

32.

Molecular markers for the diagnosis and management of ductal carcinoma in situ.

Author:	Polyak K
Institution:	Department of Medical Oncology, Dana-Farber Cancer Institute, 44 Binney St D740C, Boston, MA 02115, USA. kornelia_polyak@dfci.harvard.edu
Journal:	J Natl Cancer Inst Monogr. 2010;2010(41):210-3.
Abstract Link:	http://www.medifocus.com/abstracts.php?gid=OC008&ID=20956832

33.

Local outcomes in ductal carcinoma in situ based on patient and tumor characteristics.

Author:	Schnitt SJ
Institution:	Department of Pathology, Beth Israel Deaconess Medical Center, 330 Brookline Ave, Boston, MA 02215, USA. sschnitt@bidmc.harvard.edu
Journal:	J Natl Cancer Inst Monogr. 2010;2010(41):158-61.
Abstract Link:	http://www.medifocus.com/abstracts.php?gid=OC008&ID=20956823

34.

Association between patient and tumor characteristics with clinical outcomes in women with ductal carcinoma in situ.

Authors:	Shamliyan T; Wang SY; Virnig BA; Tuttle TM; Kane RL
Institution:	Division of Health Policy and Management, University of Minnesota School of Public Health, D330-5 Mayo (MMC 729), 420 Delaware St SE, Minneapolis, MN 55455, USA. shaml005@umn.edu
Journal:	J Natl Cancer Inst Monogr. 2010;2010(41):121-9.
Abstract Link:	http://www.medifocus.com/abstracts.php?gid=OC008&ID=20956815

35.

Sentinel lymph node biopsy and management of the axilla in ductal carcinoma in situ.

Authors:	Shapiro-Wright HM; Julian TB
Institution:	Department of Human Oncology, Allegheny General Hospital, Pittsburgh, PA 15212, USA.
Journal:	J Natl Cancer Inst Monogr. 2010;2010(41):145-9.
Abstract Link:	http://www.medifocus.com/abstracts.php?gid=OC008&ID=20956820

36.

Choosing treatment for patients with ductal carcinoma in situ: fine tuning the University of Southern California/Van Nuys Prognostic Index.

Authors:	Silverstein MJ; Lagios MD
Institution:	Breast Program, Hoag Memorial Hospital Presbyterian, Newport Beach, CA, USA. melsilver9@gmail.com
Journal:	J Natl Cancer Inst Monogr. 2010;2010(41):193-6.
Abstract Link:	http://www.medifocus.com/abstracts.php?gid=OC008&ID=20956828

Go to http://www.medifocus.com/links/OC008/0814 for direct online access to the above Abstract Links.

37.

The impact of adding radiation treatment after breast conservation surgery for ductal carcinoma in situ of the breast.

Author:	Solin LJ
Institution:	Department of Radiation Oncology, Albert Einstein Medical Center, 5501 Old York Rd, Philadelphia, PA 19141, USA. solin@einstein.edu
Journal:	J Natl Cancer Inst Monogr. 2010;2010(41):187-92.
Abstract Link:	http://www.medifocus.com/abstracts.php?gid=OC008&ID=20956827

38.

The impact of sentinel lymph node biopsy and magnetic resonance imaging on important outcomes among patients with ductal carcinoma in situ.

Authors:	Tuttle TM; Shamliyan T; Virnig BA; Kane RL
Institution:	Department of Surgery, University of Minnesota, 420 Delaware St SE, Minneapolis, MN 55455, USA. tuttl006@umn.edu
Journal:	J Natl Cancer Inst Monogr. 2010;2010(41):117-20.
Abstract Link:	http://www.medifocus.com/abstracts.php?gid=OC008&ID=20956814

39.

Ductal carcinoma in situ of the breast: a systematic review of incidence, treatment, and outcomes.

Authors:	Virnig BA; Tuttle TM; Shamliyan T; Kane RL
Institution:	Division of Health Policy and Management, University of Minnesota School of Public Health, A365 Mayo (MMC 729), Minneapolis, MN 55455, USA. virni001@umn.edu
Journal:	J Natl Cancer Inst. 2010 Feb 3;102(3):170-8. Epub 2010 Jan 13.
Abstract Link:	http://www.medifocus.com/abstracts.php?gid=OC008&ID=20071685

Go to http://www.medifocus.com/links/OC008/0814 for direct online access to the above Abstract Links.

General Interest Articles

40.

The frequency of presentation and clinico-pathological characteristics of symptomatic versus screen detected ductal carcinoma in situ of the breast.

Authors:	Barnes NL; Dimopoulos N; Williams KE; Howe M; Bundred NJ
Institution:	Array 2nd Floor, Education and Research Centre, Southmoor Road, Manchester M23 9LT, UK.
Journal:	Eur J Surg Oncol. 2014 Mar;40(3):249-54. doi: 10.1016/j.ejso.2013.12.013. Epub 2014 Jan 3.
Abstract Link:	http://www.medifocus.com/abstracts.php?gid=OC008&ID=24433818

41.

Atypical ductal hyperplasia diagnosed at sonographically guided core needle biopsy: frequency, final surgical outcome, and factors associated with underestimation.

Authors:	Mesurolle B; Perez JC; Azzumea F; Lemercier E; Xie X; Aldis A; Omeroglu A; Meterissian S
Institution:	1 All authors: Cedar Breast Clinic, McGill University Health Center, Royal Victoria Hospital, 687 Pine Ave W, Montreal, PQ, H3H 1A1 Canada.
Journal:	AJR Am J Roentgenol. 2014 Jun;202(6):1389-94. doi: 10.2214/AJR.13.10864.
Abstract Link:	http://www.medifocus.com/abstracts.php?gid=OC008&ID=24848840

Go to http://www.medifocus.com/links/OC008/0814 for direct online access to the above Abstract Links.

42.

Incidence and prediction of invasive disease and nodal metastasis in preoperatively diagnosed ductal carcinoma in situ.

Authors:	Osako T; Iwase T; Ushijima M; Horii R; Fukami Y; Kimura K; Matsuura M; Akiyama F
Institution:	Division of Pathology, The Cancer Institute of the Japanese Foundation for Cancer Research, Tokyo, Japan; Department of Pathology, The Cancer Institute Hospital of the Japanese Foundation for Cancer Research, Tokyo, Japan.
Journal:	Cancer Sci. 2014 May;105(5):576-82. doi: 10.1111/cas.12381. Epub 2014 Mar 26.
Abstract Link:	http://www.medifocus.com/abstracts.php?gid=OC008&ID=24533797

43.

Incidence of and risk factors for sentinel lymph node metastasis in patients with a postoperative diagnosis of ductal carcinoma in situ.

Authors:	Zetterlund L; Stemme S; Arnrup H; de Boniface J
Institution:	Department of Surgery, Stockholm South General Hospital, Stockholm, Sweden; Department of Clinical Science and Education, Karolinska Institute, Stockholm, Sweden.
Journal:	Br J Surg. 2014 Apr;101(5):488-94. doi: 10.1002/bjs.9404. Epub 2014 Feb 3.
Abstract Link:	http://www.medifocus.com/abstracts.php?gid=OC008&ID=24493058

44.

Impact of race and ethnicity on features and outcome of ductal carcinoma in situ of the breast.

Authors:	Bailes AA; Kuerer HM; Lari SA; Jones LA; Brewster AM
Institution:	Department of Surgical Oncology, The University of Texas M. D. Anderson Cancer Center, Houston, USA.
Journal:	Cancer. 2013 Jan 1;119(1):150-7. doi: 10.1002/cncr.27707. Epub 2012 Jun 26.
Abstract Link:	http://www.medifocus.com/abstracts.php?gid=OC008&ID=22736444

Go to http://www.medifocus.com/links/OC008/0814 for direct online access to the above Abstract Links.

45.

Psychosexual functioning and body image following a diagnosis of ductal carcinoma in situ.

Authors:	Bober SL; Giobbie-Hurder A; Emmons KM; Winer E; Partridge A
Institution:	Dana-Farber Cancer Institute, Brigham and Women's Hospital and Harvard Medical School, Boston, MA, USA. Sharon_Bober@dfci.harvard.edu
Journal:	J Sex Med. 2013 Feb;10(2):370-7. doi: 10.1111/j.1743-6109.2012.02852.x. Epub 2012 Jul 19.
Abstract Link:	http://www.medifocus.com/abstracts.php?gid=OC008&ID=22812628

46.

Tumor size, node status, grading, HER2 and estrogen receptor status still retain a strong value in patients with operable breast cancer diagnosed in recent years.

Authors:	Cortesi L; Marcheselli L; Guarneri V; Cirilli C; Braghiroli B; Toss A; Sant M; Ficarra G; Conte PF; Federico M
Institution:	Department of Oncology and Haematology, University of Modena and Reggio Emilia, Modena, Italy. hbc@unimore.it
Journal:	Int J Cancer. 2013 Jan 15;132(2):E58-65. doi: 10.1002/ijc.27795. Epub 2012 Sep 21.
Abstract Link:	http://www.medifocus.com/abstracts.php?gid=OC008&ID=22915138

47.

Risk stratification in ductal carcinoma in situ: the role of genomic testing.

Author:	Freedman GM
Institution:	Perelman School of Medicine of the University of Pennsylvania, Philadelphia, PA 19104, USA. gary.freedman@uphs.upenn.edu
Journal:	Curr Oncol Rep. 2013 Feb;15(1):7-13. doi: 10.1007/s11912-012-0280-6.
Abstract Link:	http://www.medifocus.com/abstracts.php?gid=OC008&ID=23180216

Go to http://www.medifocus.com/links/OC008/0814 for direct online access to the above Abstract Links.

48.

Nomogram for predicting invasion in patients with a preoperative diagnosis of ductal carcinoma in situ of the breast.

Authors:	Lee SK; Yang JH; Woo SY; Lee JE; Nam SJ
Institution:	Division of Breast and Endocrine Surgery, Department of Surgery, Samsung Medical Centre, Sungkyunkwan University School of Medicine, Seoul, South Korea.
Journal:	Br J Surg. 2013 Dec;100(13):1756-63. doi: 10.1002/bjs.9337.
Abstract Link:	http://www.medifocus.com/abstracts.php?gid=OC008&ID=24227361

49.

Effects of menopausal hormone therapy on ductal carcinoma in situ of the breast.

Authors:	Luo J; Cochrane BB; Wactawski-Wende J; Hunt JR; Ockene JK; Margolis KL
Institution:	Department of Epidemiology and Biostatistics, School of Public Health-Bloomington, Indiana University, Bloomington, IN, USA. juhluo@indiana.edu
Journal:	Breast Cancer Res Treat. 2013 Feb;137(3):915-25. doi: 10.1007/s10549-012-2402-0. Epub 2013 Jan 12.
Abstract Link:	http://www.medifocus.com/abstracts.php?gid=OC008&ID=23315265

50.

Intraductal therapy of ductal carcinoma in situ: a presurgery study.

Authors:	Mahoney ME; Gordon EJ; Rao JY; Jin Y; Hylton N; Love SM
Institution:	Department of Surgery, St Joseph Health, Eureka, CA, USA.
Journal:	Clin Breast Cancer. 2013 Aug;13(4):280-6. doi: 10.1016/j.clbc.2013.02.002. Epub 2013 May 9.
Abstract Link:	http://www.medifocus.com/abstracts.php?gid=OC008&ID=23664819

Go to http://www.medifocus.com/links/OC008/0814 for direct online access to the above Abstract Links.

51.

Outcomes in patients treated with mastectomy for ductal carcinoma in situ.

Authors:	Owen D; Tyldesley S; Alexander C; Speers C; Truong P; Nichol A; Wai ES
Institution:	Radiation Therapy Program, Vancouver and Victoria, British Columbia, Canada.
Journal:	Int J Radiat Oncol Biol Phys. 2013 Mar 1;85(3):e129-34. doi: 10.1016/j.ijrobp.2012.10.020. Epub 2012 Nov 27.
Abstract Link:	http://www.medifocus.com/abstracts.php?gid=OC008&ID=23195778

52.

Prediction of underestimated invasiveness in patients with ductal carcinoma in situ of the breast on percutaneous biopsy as rationale for recommending concurrent sentinel lymph node biopsy.

Authors:	Schulz S; Sinn P; Golatta M; Rauch G; Junkermann H; Schuetz F; Sohn C; Heil J
Institution:	Breast Unit, University of Heidelberg Women's Hospital, Vossstrasse 9, 69115 Heidelberg, Germany.
Journal:	Breast. 2013 Aug;22(4):537-42. doi: 10.1016/j.breast.2012.11.002. Epub 2012 Dec 11.
Abstract Link:	http://www.medifocus.com/abstracts.php?gid=OC008&ID=23237921

53.

Molecular subtypes of ductal carcinoma in situ in African American and Caucasian American women: distribution and correlation with pathological features and outcome.

Authors:	Sharaf Aldeen B; Feng J; Wu Y; Nassar Warzecha H
Institution:	Department of Pathology, Wayne State University, Detroit, MI 48201, USA. bsharafa@med.wayne.edu
Journal:	Cancer Epidemiol. 2013 Aug;37(4):474-8. doi: 10.1016/j.canep.2013.03.018. Epub 2013 Apr 30.
Abstract Link:	http://www.medifocus.com/abstracts.php?gid=OC008&ID=23639792

Go to http://www.medifocus.com/links/OC008/0814 for direct online access to the above Abstract Links.

54.

Microinvasive breast carcinoma carries an excellent prognosis regardless of the tumor characteristics.

Authors:	Shatat L; Gloyeske N; Madan R; O'Neil M; Tawfik O; Fan F
Institution:	Department of Pathology and Laboratory Medicine, University of Kansas Medical Center, Kansas City, KS 66160, USA.
Journal:	Hum Pathol. 2013 Dec;44(12):2684-9. doi: 10.1016/j.humpath.2013.07.010. Epub 2013 Sep 24.
Abstract Link:	http://www.medifocus.com/abstracts.php?gid=OC008&ID=24071019

55.

Modeling the effectiveness of initial management strategies for ductal carcinoma in situ.

Authors:	Soeteman DI; Stout NK; Ozanne EM; Greenberg C; Hassett MJ; Schrag D; Punglia RS
Institution:	Center for Health Decision Science, Department of Health Policy and Management, Harvard School of Public Health, Boston, MA 02115, USA. dsoetema@hsph.harvard.edu
Journal:	J Natl Cancer Inst. 2013 Jun 5;105(11):774-81. doi: 10.1093/jnci/djt096. Epub 2013 May 3.
Abstract Link:	http://www.medifocus.com/abstracts.php?gid=OC008&ID=23644480

56.

Does time to definitive treatment matter in patients with ductal carcinoma in situ?

Authors:	Sue GR; Lannin DR; Killelea B; Tsangaris T; Chagpar AB
Institution:	Department of Surgery, Yale University School of Medicine, New Haven, Connecticut, USA.
Journal:	Am Surg. 2013 Jun;79(6):561-5.
Abstract Link:	http://www.medifocus.com/abstracts.php?gid=OC008&ID=23711263

Go to http://www.medifocus.com/links/OC008/0814 for direct online access to the above Abstract Links.

57.

Ductal carcinoma in situ associated with triple negative invasive breast cancer: evidence for a precursor-product relationship.

Authors:	Thike AA; Iqbal J; Cheok PY; Tse GM; Tan PH
Institution:	Department of Pathology, Singapore General Hospital, Singapore.
Journal:	J Clin Pathol. 2013 Aug;66(8):665-70. doi: 10.1136/jclinpath-2012-201428. Epub 2013 Mar 28.
Abstract Link:	http://www.medifocus.com/abstracts.php?gid=OC008&ID=23539741

58.

Metastatic invasive breast cancer recurrence following curative-intent therapy for ductal carcinoma in situ.

Authors:	Al Mushawah F; Rastelli A; Pluard T; Margenthaler JA
Institution:	Department of Surgery, Washington University School of Medicine, St. Louis, Missouri 63110, USA.
Journal:	J Surg Res. 2012 Mar;173(1):10-5. Epub 2011 May 23.
Abstract Link:	http://www.medifocus.com/abstracts.php?gid=OC008&ID=21696764

59.

Should axillary ultrasound be used in patients with a preoperative diagnosis of ductal carcinoma in situ?

Authors:	Ansari B; Boughey JC; Adamczyk DL; Degnim AC; Jakub JW; Morton MJ
Institution:	Department of Surgery, Mayo Clinic, Rochester, MN, USA.
Journal:	Am J Surg. 2012 Sep;204(3):290-3. doi: 10.1016/j.amjsurg.2011.11.018. Epub 2012 Jun 30.
Abstract Link:	http://www.medifocus.com/abstracts.php?gid=OC008&ID=22749764

Go to http://www.medifocus.com/links/OC008/0814 for direct online access to the above Abstract Links.

60.

Pathologic characteristics of second breast cancers after breast conservation for ductal carcinoma in situ.

Authors:	Arvold ND; Punglia RS; Hughes ME; Jiang W; Edge SB; Javid SH; Laronga C; Niland JC; Theriault RL; Weeks JC; Wong YN; Lee SJ; Hassett MJ
Institution:	Harvard Radiation Oncology Program, Harvard Medical School, Boston, Massachusetts, USA. narvold@partners.org
Journal:	Cancer. 2012 Dec 15;118(24):6022-30. doi: 10.1002/cncr.27691. Epub 2012 Jun 6.
Abstract Link:	http://www.medifocus.com/abstracts.php?gid=OC008&ID=22674478

61.

Local recurrence rate in patients with DCIS.

Authors:	Bartova M; Suska P; Pohlodek K
Institution:	IInd Department of Gynaecology and Obstetrics, University Hospital, Bratislava, Slovakia.
Journal:	Bratisl Lek Listy. 2012;113(1):30-4.
Abstract Link:	http://www.medifocus.com/abstracts.php?gid=OC008&ID=22380499

62.

Predictive factors for BRCA1/BRCA2 mutations in women with ductal carcinoma in situ.

Authors:	Bayraktar S; Elsayegh N; Gutierrez Barrera AM; Lin H; Kuerer H; Tasbas T; Muse KI; Ready K; Litton J; Meric-Bernstam F; Hortobagyi GN; Albarracin CT; Arun B
Institution:	Division of Cancer Medicine, The University of Texas M. D. Anderson Cancer Center, Houston, Texas, USA.
Journal:	Cancer. 2012 Mar 15;118(6):1515-22. doi: 10.1002/cncr.26428. Epub 2011 Aug 25.
Abstract Link:	http://www.medifocus.com/abstracts.php?gid=OC008&ID=22009639

Go to http://www.medifocus.com/links/OC008/0814 for direct online access to the above Abstract Links.

63.

Predictive factors for breast cancer in patients diagnosed with ductal intraepithelial neoplasia, grade 1B.

Authors:	Bendifallah S; Chabbert-Buffet N; Maurin N; Chopier J; Antoine M; Bezu C; Uzan S; Rouzier R
Institution:	Department of Obstetrics and Gynecology, 4 Rue de la Chine, 75020 Paris, France. sofiane.bendifallah@yahoo.fr
Journal:	Anticancer Res. 2012 Aug;32(8):3571-9.
Abstract Link:	http://www.medifocus.com/abstracts.php?gid=OC008&ID=22843948

64.

Use of MRI in preoperative planning for women with newly diagnosed DCIS: risk or benefit?

Authors:	Davis KL; Barth RJ Jr; Gui J; Dann E; Eisenberg B; Rosenkranz K
Institution:	Department of Surgery, Dartmouth Hitchcock Medical Center, Lebanon, NH, USA.
Journal:	Ann Surg Oncol. 2012 Oct;19(10):3270-4. doi: 10.1245/s10434-012-2548-3. Epub 2012 Aug 22.
Abstract Link:	http://www.medifocus.com/abstracts.php?gid=OC008&ID=22911365

65.

HER2 evaluation and its impact on breast cancer treatment decisions.

Authors:	Goddard KA; Weinmann S; Richert-Boe K; Chen C; Bulkley J; Wax C
Institution:	The Center for Health Research, Kaiser Permanente Northwest, Portland, OR, USA. katrina.ab.goddard@kpchr.org
Journal:	Public Health Genomics. 2012;15(1):1-10. Epub 2011 May 3.
Abstract Link:	http://www.medifocus.com/abstracts.php?gid=OC008&ID=21540562

Go to http://www.medifocus.com/links/OC008/0814 for direct online access to the above Abstract Links.

66.

Evaluation of appropriate short-term mammographic surveillance in patients who undergo breast-conserving Surgery (BCS).

Authors:	Gunia SR; Merrigan TL; Poulton TB; Mamounas EP
Institution:	Affinity Medical Center, Massillon, OH, USA.
Journal:	Ann Surg Oncol. 2012 Oct;19(10):3139-43. doi: 10.1245/s10434-012-2578-x. Epub 2012 Aug 8.
Abstract Link:	http://www.medifocus.com/abstracts.php?gid=OC008&ID=22872291

67.

The shifting nature of women's experiences and perceptions of ductal carcinoma in situ.

Authors:	Kennedy F; Harcourt D; Rumsey N
Institution:	Sheffield Hallam University, UK. f.kennedy@shu.ac.uk
Journal:	J Adv Nurs. 2012 Apr;68(4):856-67. doi: 10.1111/j.1365-2648.2011.05788.x. Epub 2011 Jul 25.
Abstract Link:	http://www.medifocus.com/abstracts.php?gid=OC008&ID=21790736

68.

MRI versus breast-specific gamma imaging (BSGI) in newly diagnosed ductal cell carcinoma-in-situ: a prospective head-to-head trial.

Authors:	Keto JL; Kirstein L; Sanchez DP; Fulop T; McPartland L; Cohen I; Boolbol SK
Institution:	Department of Surgery, Beth Israel Medical Center, New York, NY, USA.
Journal:	Ann Surg Oncol. 2012 Jan;19(1):249-52. Epub 2011 Jul 8.
Abstract Link:	http://www.medifocus.com/abstracts.php?gid=OC008&ID=21739318

Go to http://www.medifocus.com/links/OC008/0814 for direct online access to the above Abstract Links.

69.

Factors associated with upstaging from ductal carcinoma in situ following core needle biopsy to invasive cancer in subsequent surgical excision.

Authors:	Kim J; Han W; Lee JW; You JM; Shin HC; Ahn SK; Moon HG; Cho N; Moon WK; Park IA; Noh DY
Institution:	Department of Surgery, Seoul National University College of Medicine, Seoul, Republic of Korea.
Journal:	Breast. 2012 Oct;21(5):641-5. doi: 10.1016/j.breast.2012.06.012. Epub 2012 Jun 30.
Abstract Link:	http://www.medifocus.com/abstracts.php?gid=OC008&ID=22749854

70.

The value of mammography within 1 year of conservative surgery for breast cancer.

Authors:	Lewis JL; Tartter PI
Institution:	St. Luke's-Roosevelt Hospital Center, New York, NY, USA. janalew@gmail.com
Journal:	Ann Surg Oncol. 2012 Oct;19(10):3218-22. doi: 10.1245/s10434-012-2480-6. Epub 2012 Jul 6.
Abstract Link:	http://www.medifocus.com/abstracts.php?gid=OC008&ID=22766990

71.

Atypical ductal hyperplasia on core biopsy: an automatic trigger for excisional biopsy?

Authors:	McGhan LJ; Pockaj BA; Wasif N; Giurescu ME; McCullough AE; Gray RJ
Institution:	Section of Surgical Oncology, Department of Surgery, Mayo Clinic Hospital, Mayo Clinic, Phoenix, AZ, USA.
Journal:	Ann Surg Oncol. 2012 Oct;19(10):3264-9. doi: 10.1245/s10434-012-2575-0. Epub 2012 Aug 10.
Abstract Link:	http://www.medifocus.com/abstracts.php?gid=OC008&ID=22878619

Go to http://www.medifocus.com/links/OC008/0814 for direct online access to the above Abstract Links.

72.

Outcome of patients with ductal carcinoma in situ and sentinel node biopsy.

Authors:	Meretoja TJ; Heikkila PS; Salmenkivi K; Leidenius MH
Institution:	Breast Surgery Unit, Department of Gastrointestinal and General Surgery, Helsinki University Central Hospital, Helsinki, Finland. tuomo.meretoja@fimnet.fi
Journal:	Ann Surg Oncol. 2012 Jul;19(7):2345-51. doi: 10.1245/s10434-012-2287-5. Epub 2012 Mar 7.
Abstract Link:	http://www.medifocus.com/abstracts.php?gid=OC008&ID=22395995

73.

Identification of copy number alterations associated with the progression of DCIS to invasive ductal carcinoma.

Authors:	O'Suilleabhain, Padraig E; Dewey, Richard B Jr; Johnson CE; Gorringe KL; Thompson ER; Opeskin K; Boyle SE; Wang Y; Hill P; Mann GB; Campbell IG
Institution:	VBCRC Cancer Genetics Laboratory, Peter MacCallum Cancer Centre, Locked Bag 1, A'Beckett St, East Melbourne, Victoria, VIC 8006, Australia.
Journal:	Breast Cancer Res Treat. 2012 Jun;133(3):889-98. doi: 10.1007/s10549-011-1835-1. Epub 2011 Nov 4.
Abstract Link:	http://www.medifocus.com/abstracts.php?gid=OC008&ID=22052326

74.

Ductal carcinoma in situ with microinvasion: prognostic implications, long-term outcomes, and role of axillary evaluation.

Authors:	Parikh RR; Haffty BG; Lannin D; Moran MS
Institution:	The Cancer Institute of New Jersey, University of Medicine and Dentistry, New Jersey-Robert Wood Johnson Medical School, New Brunswick, NJ, USA.
Journal:	Int J Radiat Oncol Biol Phys. 2012 Jan 1;82(1):7-13. Epub 2010 Oct 13.
Abstract Link:	http://www.medifocus.com/abstracts.php?gid=OC008&ID=20950955

Go to http://www.medifocus.com/links/OC008/0814 for direct online access to the above Abstract Links.

75.

HER2/neu and Ki-67 expression predict non-invasive recurrence following breast-conserving therapy for ductal carcinoma in situ.

Authors:	Rakovitch E; Nofech-Mozes S; Hanna W; Narod S; Thiruchelvam D; Saskin R; Spayne J; Taylor C; Paszat L
Institution:	Department of Radiation Oncology, University of Toronto, Toronto, Canada. eileen.rakovitch@sunnybrook.ca
Journal:	Br J Cancer. 2012 Mar 13;106(6):1160-5. doi: 10.1038/bjc.2012.41. Epub 2012 Feb 23.
Abstract Link:	http://www.medifocus.com/abstracts.php?gid=OC008&ID=22361634

76.

Comparison of the effects of genetic and environmental risk factors on in situ and invasive ductal breast cancer.

Authors:	Reeves GK; Pirie K; Green J; Bull D; Beral V
Institution:	University of Oxford, Oxford, UK. gill.reeves@ceu.ox.ac.uk
Journal:	Int J Cancer. 2012 Aug 15;131(4):930-7. doi: 10.1002/ijc.26460. Epub 2011 Nov 28.
Abstract Link:	http://www.medifocus.com/abstracts.php?gid=OC008&ID=21952983

77.

Risk factor for axillary lymph node metastases in microinvasive breast cancer.

Authors:	Schweiger LM.; Hsiang HY.; Ko BS; Lim WS; Kim HJ; Yu JH; Lee JW; Kwan SB; Lee YM; Son BH; Gong GY; Ahn SH
Institution:	Department of Surgery, Asan Medical Center, University of Ulsan, College of Medicine, Seoul, Korea.
Journal:	Ann Surg Oncol. 2012 Jan;19(1):212-6. Epub 2011 Jun 2.
Abstract Link:	http://www.medifocus.com/abstracts.php?gid=OC008&ID=21633867

Go to http://www.medifocus.com/links/OC008/0814 for direct online access to the above Abstract Links.

78.

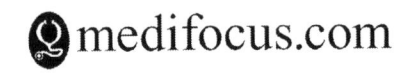

Predictors of invasive breast cancer and lymph node involvement in ductal carcinoma in situ initially diagnosed by vacuum-assisted breast biopsy: experience of 733 cases.

Authors:	Trentin C; Dominelli V; Maisonneuve P; Menna S; Bazolli B; Luini A; Cassano E
Institution:	Division of Breast Radiology, European Institute of Oncology, Via Ripamonti 435, Milan, Italy. chiara.trentin@ieo.it
Journal:	Breast. 2012 Oct;21(5):635-40. doi: 10.1016/j.breast.2012.06.009. Epub 2012 Jul 12.
Abstract Link:	http://www.medifocus.com/abstracts.php?gid=OC008&ID=22795363

79.

The effect of DCIS grade on rate, type and time to recurrence after 15 years of follow-up of screen-detected DCIS.

Authors:	Wallis MG; Clements K; Kearins O; Ball G; Macartney J; Lawrence GM
Institution:	Cambridge Breast Unit and NIHR Cambridge Biomedical Research Unit, Box 97, Cambridge University Hospitals NHS Foundation Trust, Hills Road, Cambridge CB2 0QQ, UK. matthew.wallis@addenbrookes.nhs.uk
Journal:	Br J Cancer. 2012 May 8;106(10):1611-7. doi: 10.1038/bjc.2012.151. Epub 2012 Apr 19.
Abstract Link:	http://www.medifocus.com/abstracts.php?gid=OC008&ID=22516949

80.

Evaluation of a breast cancer nomogram for predicting risk of ipsilateral breast tumor recurrences in patients with ductal carcinoma in situ after local excision.

Authors:	Yi M; Meric-Bernstam F; Kuerer HM; Mittendorf EA; Bedrosian I; Lucci A; Hwang RF; Crow JR; Luo S; Hunt KK
Institution:	Department of Surgical Oncology, Unit 1484, The University of Texas MD Anderson Cancer Center, 1400 Pressler St, Houston, TX 77030, USA.
Journal:	J Clin Oncol. 2012 Feb 20;30(6):600-7. Epub 2012 Jan 17.

Go to http://www.medifocus.com/links/OC008/0814 for direct online access to the above Abstract Links.

Abstract Link: http://www.medifocus.com/abstracts.php?gid=OC008&ID=22253459

81.

Fine tuning of the Van Nuys prognostic index (VNPI) 2003 by integrating the genomic grade index (GGI): new tools for ductal carcinoma in situ (DCIS).

Authors:	Altintas S; Toussaint J; Durbecq V; Lambein K; Huizing MT; Larsimont D; Van Marck E; Vermorken JB; Tjalma WA; Sotiriou C
Institution:	Department of Medical Oncology, Antwerp University Hospital, Edegem, Belgium. sevilay.altintas@uza.be
Journal:	Breast J. 2011 Jul-Aug;17(4):343-51. doi: 10.1111/j.1524-4741.2011.01091.x. Epub 2011 Jun 6.
Abstract Link:	http://www.medifocus.com/abstracts.php?gid=OC008&ID=21645166

82.

Molecular subtyping of DCIS: heterogeneity of breast cancer reflected in pre-invasive disease.

Authors:	Clark SE; Warwick J; Carpenter R; Bowen RL; Duffy SW; Jones JL
Institution:	Centre for Tumour Biology, Institute of Cancer and CR-UK Clinical Centre, Barts and the London School of Medicine and Dentistry, John Vane Science Centre, Charterhouse Square, London EC1M 6BQ, UK. sarahclark74@hotmail.com
Journal:	Br J Cancer. 2011 Jan 4;104(1):120-7. Epub 2010 Dec 7.
Abstract Link:	http://www.medifocus.com/abstracts.php?gid=OC008&ID=21139586

83.

Understanding a ductal carcinoma in situ diagnosis: patient views and surgeon descriptions.

Authors:	Davey C; White V; Warne C; Kitchen P; Villanueva E; Erbas B
Institution:	Centre for Behavioural Research in Cancer, The Cancer Council Victoria, Carlton, Victoria, Australia.
Journal:	Eur J Cancer Care (Engl). 2011 Nov;20(6):776-84. doi: 10.1111/j.1365-2354.2011.01265.x. Epub 2011 Jul 19.
Abstract Link:	http://www.medifocus.com/abstracts.php?gid=OC008&ID=21771131

Go to http://www.medifocus.com/links/OC008/0814 for direct online access to the above Abstract Links.

84.

Digital mammography screening: weighing reduced mortality against increased overdiagnosis.

Authors:	de Gelder R; Fracheboud J; Heijnsdijk EA; den Heeten G; Verbeek AL; Broeders MJ; Draisma G; de Koning HJ
Institution:	Erasmus MC, Department of Public Health, P.O. Box 2040, 3000 CA, Rotterdam, The Netherlands. r.degelder@erasmusmc.nl
Journal:	Prev Med. 2011 Sep 1;53(3):134-40. Epub 2011 Jun 21.
Abstract Link:	http://www.medifocus.com/abstracts.php?gid=OC008&ID=21718717

85.

Knowledge, satisfaction with information, decisional conflict and psychological morbidity amongst women diagnosed with ductal carcinoma in situ (DCIS).

Authors:	De Morgan S; Redman S; D'Este C; Rogers K
Institution:	Faculty of Behavioural Science in Relation to Medicine, University of Newcastle, Newcastle, Australia. simoned@ihug.com.au
Journal:	Patient Educ Couns. 2011 Jul;84(1):62-8. Epub 2010 Aug 9.
Abstract Link:	http://www.medifocus.com/abstracts.php?gid=OC008&ID=20696544

86.

What is the malignant nature of human ductal carcinoma in situ?

Authors:	Espina V; Liotta LA
Institution:	George Mason University, Center for Applied Proteomics and Molecular Medicine, Manassas, Virginia 20110, USA.
Journal:	Nat Rev Cancer. 2011 Jan;11(1):68-75. Epub 2010 Dec 2.
Abstract Link:	http://www.medifocus.com/abstracts.php?gid=OC008&ID=21150936

87.

The management of ductal intraepithelial neoplasia (DIN): open controversies and guidelines of the Istituto Europeo di Oncologia (IEO), Milan, Italy.

Authors:	Farante G; Zurrida S; Galimberti V; Veronesi P; Curigliano G; Luini A; Goldhirsch A; Veronesi U
Institution:	Division of Senology, European Institute of Oncology, IEO, Via Ripamonti 435, 20141 Milan, Italy. gabriel.farante@ieo.it
Journal:	Breast Cancer Res Treat. 2011 Jul;128(2):369-78. Epub 2010 Aug 26.
Abstract Link:	http://www.medifocus.com/abstracts.php?gid=OC008&ID=20740312

88.

The significance of HER-2/neu receptor positivity and immunophenotype in ductal carcinoma in situ with early invasive disease.

Authors:	Harada S; Mick R; Roses RE; Graves H; Niu H; Sharma A; Schueller JE; Nisenbaum H; Czerniecki BJ; Zhang PJ
Institution:	Department of Pathology and Laboratory Medicine, The University of Pennsylvania, Philadelphia, Pennsylvania, USA.
Journal:	J Surg Oncol. 2011 Oct;104(5):458-65. doi: 10.1002/jso.21973. Epub 2011 May 9.
Abstract Link:	http://www.medifocus.com/abstracts.php?gid=OC008&ID=21557226

89.

The effect of age in the outcome and treatment of older women with ductal carcinoma in situ.

Authors:	Ho A; Goenka A; Ishill N; Van Zee K; McLane A; Gonzales AM; Tan L; Cody H; Powell S; McCormick B
Institution:	Department of Radiation Oncology, Memorial Sloan-Kettering Cancer Center, 1275 York Avenue, New York, NY, USA. hoa1234@mskcc.org
Journal:	Breast. 2011 Feb;20(1):71-7. Epub 2010 Aug 23.
Abstract Link:	http://www.medifocus.com/abstracts.php?gid=OC008&ID=20739181

Go to http://www.medifocus.com/links/OC008/0814 for direct online access to the above Abstract Links.

90.

Prognostic markers and long-term outcomes in ductal carcinoma in situ of the breast treated with excision alone.

Authors:	Holmes P; Lloyd J; Chervoneva I; Pequinot E; Cornfield DB; Schwartz GF; Allen KG; Palazzo JP
Institution:	Department of Pathology, Anatomy, and Cell Biology, Thomas Jefferson University Hospital, Philadelphia, Pennsylvania, USA.
Journal:	Cancer. 2011 Aug 15;117(16):3650-7. doi: 10.1002/cncr.25942. Epub 2011 Feb 11.
Abstract Link:	http://www.medifocus.com/abstracts.php?gid=OC008&ID=21319154

91.

Update on DCIS outcomes from the American Society of Breast Surgeons accelerated partial breast irradiation registry trial.

Authors:	Jeruss JS; Kuerer HM; Beitsch PD; Vicini FA; Keisch M
Institution:	Department of Surgery, Northwestern University Feinberg School of Medicine, Chicago, IL, USA. jjeruss@nmh.org
Journal:	Ann Surg Oncol. 2011 Jan;18(1):65-71. Epub 2010 Jun 25.
Abstract Link:	http://www.medifocus.com/abstracts.php?gid=OC008&ID=20577822

92.

HER2-positive status is an independent predictor for coexisting invasion of ductal carcinoma in situ of the breast presenting extensive DCIS component.

Authors:	Liao N; Zhang GC; Liu YH; Li XR; Yao M; Xu FP; Li L; Wu YL
Institution:	Southern Medical University, Guangzhou, China.
Journal:	Pathol Res Pract. 2011 Jan 15;207(1):1-7. Epub 2010 Nov 20.
Abstract Link:	http://www.medifocus.com/abstracts.php?gid=OC008&ID=21095069

Go to http://www.medifocus.com/links/OC008/0814 for direct online access to the above Abstract Links.

93.

Indication for sentinel lymph node biopsy for breast cancer when core biopsy shows ductal carcinoma in situ.

Authors:	Miyake T; Shimazu K; Ohashi H; Taguchi T; Ueda S; Nakayama T; Kim SJ; Aozasa K; Tamaki Y; Noguchi S
Institution:	Department of Breast and Endocrine Surgery, Osaka University, Graduate School of Medicine, Suita, Japan.
Journal:	Am J Surg. 2011 Jul;202(1):59-65.
Abstract Link:	http://www.medifocus.com/abstracts.php?gid=OC008&ID=21741518

94.

Ductal carcinoma-in-situ of the breast with subsequent distant metastasis and death.

Authors:	Roses RE; Arun BK; Lari SA; Mittendorf EA; Lucci A; Hunt KK; Kuerer HM
Institution:	Department of Surgical Oncology, The University of Texas M. D. Anderson Cancer Center, Houston, TX, USA.
Journal:	Ann Surg Oncol. 2011 Oct;18(10):2873-8. Epub 2011 Apr 8.
Abstract Link:	http://www.medifocus.com/abstracts.php?gid=OC008&ID=21476105

95.

Can we know what to do when DCIS is diagnosed?

Authors:	Sanders ME; Simpson JF
Institution:	Department of Pathology, Vanderbilt University School of Medicine, Nashville, Tennessee 37232, USA.
Journal:	Oncology (Williston Park). 2011 Aug;25(9):852-6.
Abstract Link:	http://www.medifocus.com/abstracts.php?gid=OC008&ID=21936451

Go to http://www.medifocus.com/links/OC008/0814 for direct online access to the above Abstract Links.

96.

Disseminated tumor cells in the bone marrow of patients with ductal carcinoma in situ.

Authors:	Sanger N; Effenberger KE; Riethdorf S; Van Haasteren V; Gauwerky J; Wiegratz I; Strebhardt K; Kaufmann M; Pantel K
Institution:	Department of Gynaecology and Obstetrics, University Hospital Frankfurt, Frankfurt, Germany.
Journal:	Int J Cancer. 2011 Nov 15;129(10):2522-6. doi: 10.1002/ijc.25895. Epub 2011 Mar 25.
Abstract Link:	http://www.medifocus.com/abstracts.php?gid=OC008&ID=21207426

97.

Premalignant lesions: diagnosis, evaluation, and management.

Author:	Tejada-Berges T
Institution:	The Warren Alpert School of Medicine of Brown University, Department of Obstetrics and Gynecology, Program in Women's Oncology, Women and Infants' Hospital, Providence, Rhode Island, USA. ttejadaberges@wihri.org
Journal:	Clin Obstet Gynecol. 2011 Mar;54(1):133-40.
Abstract Link:	http://www.medifocus.com/abstracts.php?gid=OC008&ID=21278512

98.

Ductal carcinoma in situ of the breast: influence of age on diagnostic, therapeutic, and prognostic features. Retrospective study of 812 patients.

Authors:	Tunon-de-Lara C; Andre G; Macgrogan G; Dilhuydy JM; Bussieres JE; Debled M; Mauriac L; Brouste V; de Mascarel I; Avril A
Institution:	Department of Surgery, Institut Bergonie, Bordeaux Cedex, France. tunon@bergonie.org
Journal:	Ann Surg Oncol. 2011 May;18(5):1372-9. Epub 2010 Nov 25.
Abstract Link:	http://www.medifocus.com/abstracts.php?gid=OC008&ID=21108045

Go to http://www.medifocus.com/links/OC008/0814 for direct online access to the above Abstract Links.

99.

Selective approach to radionuclide-guided sentinel lymph node biopsy in high-risk ductal carcinoma in situ of the breast.

Authors:	Usmani S; Khan HA; Al Saleh N; abu Huda F; Marafi F; Amanguno HG; Al Nafisi N; Al Kandari F
Institution:	Department of Nuclear Medicine, Hussain Makki Al Jumma Centre for Specialized Surgery, Khaitan, Kuwait. dr_shajji@yahoo.com
Journal:	Nucl Med Commun. 2011 Nov;32(11):1084-7.
Abstract Link:	http://www.medifocus.com/abstracts.php?gid=OC008&ID=21862942

100.

Ductal carcinoma in situ: trends in treatment over time in the US.

Authors:	Zujewski JA; Harlan LC; Morrell DM; Stevens JL
Institution:	National Cancer Institute, CTEP, Bethesda, MD, USA.
Journal:	Breast Cancer Res Treat. 2011 May;127(1):251-7. Epub 2010 Oct 8.
Abstract Link:	http://www.medifocus.com/abstracts.php?gid=OC008&ID=20931276

101.

National Institutes of Health State-of-the-Science Conference statement: Diagnosis and Management of Ductal Carcinoma In Situ September 22-24, 2009.

Authors:	Allegra CJ; Aberle DR; Ganschow P; Hahn SM; Lee CN; Millon-Underwood S; Pike MC; Reed SD; Saftlas AF; Scarvalone SA; Schwartz AM; Slomski C; Yothers G; Zon R
Institution:	University of Florida Shands Cancer Center, Department of Medicine, University of Florida, Gainesville, FL 32610, USA. carmen.allegra@medicine.ufl.edu
Journal:	J Natl Cancer Inst. 2010 Feb 3;102(3):161-9. Epub 2010 Jan 13.
Abstract Link:	http://www.medifocus.com/abstracts.php?gid=OC008&ID=20071686

Go to http://www.medifocus.com/links/OC008/0814 for direct online access to the above Abstract Links.

102.

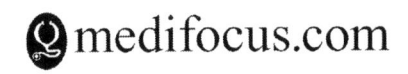

Risk reduction strategies for ductal carcinoma in situ.

Authors:	Cohen AL; Ward JH
Institution:	Oncology Division, Department of Internal Medicine, University of Utah School of Medicine, Salt Lake City, Utah 84112-5550, USA.
Journal:	J Natl Compr Canc Netw. 2010 Oct;8(10):1211-7.
Abstract Link:	http://www.medifocus.com/abstracts.php?gid=OC008&ID=20971843

103.

The role of socioeconomic status in adjustment after ductal carcinoma in situ.

Authors:	de Moor JS; Partridge AH; Winer EP; Ligibel J; Emmons KM
Institution:	the Ohio State University College of Public Health, Columbus, Ohio, USA. jdemoor@cph.osu.edu
Journal:	Cancer. 2010 Mar 1;116(5):1218-25.
Abstract Link:	http://www.medifocus.com/abstracts.php?gid=OC008&ID=20143325

104.

The psychosocial impact of ductal carcinoma in situ (DCIS): a longitudinal prospective study.

Authors:	Kennedy F; Harcourt D; Rumsey N; White P
Institution:	Centre for Appearance Research, Faculty of Health and Life Sciences, University of the West of England, Bristol, United Kingdom. F.Kennedy@shu.ac.uk
Journal:	Breast. 2010 Oct;19(5):382-7. Epub 2010 Apr 21.
Abstract Link:	http://www.medifocus.com/abstracts.php?gid=OC008&ID=20413310

Go to http://www.medifocus.com/links/OC008/0814 for direct online access to the above Abstract Links.

105.

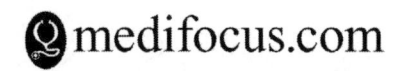

Biomarker expression and risk of subsequent tumors after initial ductal carcinoma in situ diagnosis.

Authors:	Kerlikowske K; Molinaro AM; Gauthier ML; Berman HK; Waldman F; Bennington J; Sanchez H; Jimenez C; Stewart K; Chew K; Ljung BM; Tlsty TD
Institution:	University of California, San Francisco, CA 94121, USA. karla.kerlikowkse@ucsf.edu
Journal:	J Natl Cancer Inst. 2010 May 5;102(9):627-37. Epub 2010 Apr 28.
Abstract Link:	http://www.medifocus.com/abstracts.php?gid=OC008&ID=20427430

106.

Psychological distress and physical health in the year after diagnosis of DCIS or invasive breast cancer.

Authors:	Lauzier S; Maunsell E; Levesque P; Mondor M; Robert J; Robidoux A; Provencher L
Institution:	Unite de recherche en sante des populations, Hopital du Saint-Sacrement, Centre de recherche du Centre hospitalier affile universitaire de Quebec, 1050 chemin Sainte-Foy, Quebec, QC, G1S 4L8, Canada.
Journal:	Breast Cancer Res Treat. 2010 Apr;120(3):685-91. Epub 2009 Aug 4.
Abstract Link:	http://www.medifocus.com/abstracts.php?gid=OC008&ID=19653097

107.

Ductal carcinoma in situ: size and resection volume predict margin status.

Authors:	Melstrom LG; Melstrom KA; Wang EC; Pilewskie M; Winchester DJ
Institution:	Department of Surgery, Northwestern University, Chicago, IL, USA.
Journal:	Am J Clin Oncol. 2010 Oct;33(5):438-42.
Abstract Link:	http://www.medifocus.com/abstracts.php?gid=OC008&ID=20023569

Go to http://www.medifocus.com/links/OC008/0814 for direct online access to the above Abstract Links.

108.

Ductal carcinoma in situ of the breast. Long-term follow-up of health-related quality of life, emotional reactions and body image.

Authors:	Sackey H; Sandelin K; Frisell J; Wickman M; Brandberg Y
Institution:	Department of Molecular Medicine and Surgery, Karolinska Institutet, Karolinska University Hospital, P9:03, 171 76 Stockholm, Sweden. helena.sackey@ki.se
Journal:	Eur J Surg Oncol. 2010 Aug;36(8):756-62. Epub 2010 Jul 3.
Abstract Link:	http://www.medifocus.com/abstracts.php?gid=OC008&ID=20598492

109.

The use of sentinel lymph node biopsy in ductal carcinoma in situ.

Authors:	Schneider C; Trocha S; McKinley B; Shaw J; Bielby S; Blackhurst D; Jones Y; Cornett W
Institution:	Greenville Hospital System University Medical Center, Department of Surgery, Greenville, South Carolina 29605, USA. cschneider@ghs.org
Journal:	Am Surg. 2010 Sep;76(9):943-6.
Abstract Link:	http://www.medifocus.com/abstracts.php?gid=OC008&ID=20836339

110.

Prognostic significance of HER-2/neu expression in patients with ductal carcinoma in situ.

Authors:	Stackievicz R; Paran H; Bernheim J; Shapira M; Weisenberg N; Kaufman T; Klein E; Gutman M
Institution:	Department of Diagnostic Imaging, Meir Medical Center, Kfar Saba, Israel.
Journal:	Isr Med Assoc J. 2010 May;12(5):290-5.
Abstract Link:	http://www.medifocus.com/abstracts.php?gid=OC008&ID=20929083

Go to http://www.medifocus.com/links/OC008/0814 for direct online access to the above Abstract Links.

111.

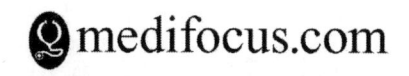

Ductal carcinoma in situ and sentinel lymph node metastasis in breast cancer.

Authors:	Tada K; Ogiya A; Kimura K; Morizono H; Iijima K; Miyagi Y; Nishimura S; Makita M; Horii R; Akiyama F; Iwase T
Institution:	Department of Breast Surgery, Cancer Institute Hospital, Tokyo, Japan. ktada@jfcr.or.jp
Journal:	World J Surg Oncol. 2010 Jan 27;8:6.
Abstract Link:	http://www.medifocus.com/abstracts.php?gid=OC008&ID=20105298

112.

Microinvasive ductal carcinoma in situ: clinical presentation, imaging features, pathologic findings, and outcome.

Authors:	Vieira CC; Mercado CL; Cangiarella JF; Moy L; Toth HK; Guth AA
Institution:	Department of Radiology, New York University School of Medicine, United States.
Journal:	Eur J Radiol. 2010 Jan;73(1):102-7. Epub 2008 Nov 21.
Abstract Link:	http://www.medifocus.com/abstracts.php?gid=OC008&ID=19026501

113.

Long-term survival of women with basal-like ductal carcinoma in situ of the breast: a population-based cohort study.

Authors:	Zhou W; Jirstrom K; Johansson C; Amini RM; Blomqvist C; Agbaje O; Warnberg F
Institution:	Department of Surgical Science, Uppsala University, Uppsala, SE-75105, Sweden. wenjing.zhou@surgsci.uu.se
Journal:	BMC Cancer. 2010 Nov 30;10:653.
Abstract Link:	http://www.medifocus.com/abstracts.php?gid=OC008&ID=21118480

Go to http://www.medifocus.com/links/OC008/0814 for direct online access to the above Abstract Links.

Drug Therapy Articles

114.

Adjuvant tamoxifen reduces subsequent breast cancer in women with estrogen receptor-positive ductal carcinoma in situ: a study based on NSABP protocol B-24.

Authors:	Allred DC; Anderson SJ; Paik S; Wickerham DL; Nagtegaal ID; Swain SM; Mamounas EP; Julian TB; Geyer CE Jr; Costantino JP; Land SR; Wolmark N
Institution:	National Surgical Adjuvant Breast and Bowel Project, Washington University School of Medicine, Department of Pathology and Immunology, 660 Euclid Campus Box 8118, St Louis, MO 63110, USA. dcallred@path.wustl.edu
Journal:	J Clin Oncol. 2012 Apr 20;30(12):1268-73. Epub 2012 Mar 5.
Abstract Link:	http://www.medifocus.com/abstracts.php?gid=OC008&ID=22393101

115.

Tamoxifen added to radiotherapy and surgery for the treatment of ductal carcinoma in situ of the breast: a meta-analysis of 2 randomized trials.

Authors:	Petrelli F; Barni S
Institution:	Azienda Ospedaliera Treviglio-Caravaggio, BG, Italy. faupe@libero.it
Journal:	Radiother Oncol. 2011 Aug;100(2):195-9. Epub 2011 Mar 14.
Abstract Link:	http://www.medifocus.com/abstracts.php?gid=OC008&ID=21411161

Surgical Therapy Articles

116.

Sentinel lymph node biopsy during prophylactic mastectomy: is there a role?

Authors:	Bunting PW; Cyr AE; Gao F; Margenthaler JA
Institution:	Department of Surgery, Washington University School of Medicine, St. Louis, Missouri.
Journal:	J Surg Oncol. 2014 Jun;109(8):747-50. doi: 10.1002/jso.23575. Epub 2014 Feb 17.
Abstract Link:	http://www.medifocus.com/abstracts.php?gid=OC008&ID=24535940

117.

Characteristics associated with upgrading to invasiveness after surgery of a DCIS diagnosed using percutaneous biopsy.

Authors:	Hogue JC; Morais L; Provencher L; Desbiens C; Poirier B; Poirier E; Jacob S; Diorio C
Institution:	Oncology Research Unit, CHU de Quebec Research Centre, 1050 chemin Ste-Foy, Quebec City, QC, Canada, G1S 4L8. caroline.diorio@uresp.ulaval.ca.
Journal:	Anticancer Res. 2014 Mar;34(3):1183-91.
Abstract Link:	http://www.medifocus.com/abstracts.php?gid=OC008&ID=24596358

118.

Impact of atypical hyperplasia at margins of breast-conserving surgery on the recurrence of breast cancer.

Authors:	Li S; Liu J; Yang Y; Zeng Y; Deng H; Jia H; Li Q; Feng H; Li Y; Song E; Liu Q; Su F
Institution:	Breast Tumor Center, Sun Yat-Sen Memorial Hospital, 33 Yingfeng Road, Guangzhou, 510288, China.
Journal:	J Cancer Res Clin Oncol. 2014 Apr;140(4):599-605. doi: 10.1007/s00432-014-1597-3. Epub 2014 Feb 9.
Abstract Link:	http://www.medifocus.com/abstracts.php?gid=OC008&ID=24509653

Go to http://www.medifocus.com/links/OC008/0814 for direct online access to the above Abstract Links.

119.

Outcomes of low-risk ductal carcinoma in situ in Southeast Asian women treated with breast conservation therapy.

Authors:	Wong FY; Wang F; Chen JJ; Tan CH; Tan PH
Institution:	Department of Radiation Oncology, National Cancer Centre Singapore, Singapore. Electronic address: fuhyong@yahoo.com.; Department of Radiation Oncology, National Cancer Centre Singapore, Singapore.; Department of Cancer Informatics, National Cancer Centre Singapore, Singapore.; Department of Radiation Oncology, National Cancer Centre Singapore, Singapore.; Department of Pathology, Singapore General Hospital, Singapore.
Journal:	Int J Radiat Oncol Biol Phys. 2014 Apr 1;88(5):998-1003. doi: 10.1016/j.ijrobp.2014.01.018.
Abstract Link:	http://www.medifocus.com/abstracts.php?gid=OC008&ID=24661651

120.

Impact of margin status on local recurrence after mastectomy for ductal carcinoma in situ.

Authors:	Childs SK; Chen YH; Duggan MM; Golshan M; Pochebit S; Punglia RS; Wong JS; Bellon JR
Institution:	Harvard Radiation Oncology Program, Boston, MA 02115, USA.
Journal:	Int J Radiat Oncol Biol Phys. 2013 Mar 15;85(4):948-52. doi: 10.1016/j.ijrobp.2012.07.2377. Epub 2012 Sep 11.
Abstract Link:	http://www.medifocus.com/abstracts.php?gid=OC008&ID=22975615

121.

Improved outcomes of breast-conserving therapy for patients with ductal carcinoma in situ.

Authors:	Halasz LM; Sreedhara M; Chen YH; Bellon JR; Punglia RS; Wong JS; Harris JR; Brock JE
Institution:	Harvard Radiation Oncology Program, Boston, MA, USA.
Journal:	Int J Radiat Oncol Biol Phys. 2012 Mar 15;82(4):e581-6. Epub 2011 Dec 28.
Abstract Link:	http://www.medifocus.com/abstracts.php?gid=OC008&ID=22208975

122.

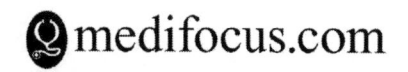

Indication for relumpectomy--a useful scoring system in cases of invasive breast cancer.

Authors:	Halevy A; Lavy R; Pappo I; Davidson T; Gold-Deutch R; Jeroukhimov I; Shapira Z; Wassermann I; Sandbank J; Chikman B
Institution:	Division of Surgery, Assaf Harofeh Medical Center, Zerifin, Israel. ahalevi@asaf.health.gov.il
Journal:	J Surg Oncol. 2012 Mar 15;105(4):376-80. doi: 10.1002/jso.22027. Epub 2011 Jul 20.
Abstract Link:	http://www.medifocus.com/abstracts.php?gid=OC008&ID=21780127

123.

Clinical outcomes of ductal carcinoma in situ of the breast treated with partial mastectomy without adjuvant radiotherapy.

Authors:	Hwang SH; Jeong J; Ahn SG; Lee HM; Lee HD
Institution:	Breast Cancer Center, Department of Surgery, Gangnam Severance Hospital, Yonsei University College of Medicine, 211 Eonju-ro, Gangnam-gu, Seoul 135-720, Korea.
Journal:	Yonsei Med J. 2012 May;53(3):537-42. doi: 10.3349/ymj.2012.53.3.537.
Abstract Link:	http://www.medifocus.com/abstracts.php?gid=OC008&ID=22476997

124.

Surgical delay of the nipple-areolar complex: a powerful technique to maximize nipple viability following nipple-sparing mastectomy.

Authors:	Jensen JA; Lin JH; Kapoor N; Giuliano AE
Institution:	Division of Plastic Surgery, Geffen School of Medicine at U.C.L.A., Los Angeles, CA, USA. Dr.J.Jensen@gmail.com
Journal:	Ann Surg Oncol. 2012 Oct;19(10):3171-6. doi: 10.1245/s10434-012-2528-7. Epub 2012 Jul 25.
Abstract Link:	http://www.medifocus.com/abstracts.php?gid=OC008&ID=22829005

Go to http://www.medifocus.com/links/OC008/0814 for direct online access to the above Abstract Links.

125.

Utilization of lymph node assessment in patients with ductal carcinoma in situ treated with lumpectomy.

Authors:	Shah DR; Canter RJ; Khatri VP; Bold RJ; Martinez SR
Institution:	Department of Surgery, Division of Surgical Oncology, University of California Davis, Sacramento, California, USA.
Journal:	J Surg Res. 2012 Sep;177(1):e21-6. doi: 10.1016/j.jss.2012.03.015. Epub 2012 Mar 30.
Abstract Link:	http://www.medifocus.com/abstracts.php?gid=OC008&ID=22482771

126.

Long-term outcome in patients with ductal carcinoma in situ treated with breast-conserving therapy: implications for optimal follow-up strategies.

Authors:	Shaitelman SF; Wilkinson JB; Kestin LL; Ye H; Goldstein NS; Martinez AA; Vicini FA
Institution:	Department of Radiation Oncology, The University of Texas MD Anderson Cancer Center, Houston, Texas, USA.
Journal:	Int J Radiat Oncol Biol Phys. 2012 Jul 1;83(3):e305-12. doi: 10.1016/j.ijrobp.2011.12.092. Epub 2012 Mar 13.
Abstract Link:	http://www.medifocus.com/abstracts.php?gid=OC008&ID=22417804

127.

Prospective evaluation of the nipple-areola complex sparing mastectomy for risk reduction and for early-stage breast cancer.

Authors:	Wagner JL; Fearmonti R; Hunt KK; Hwang RF; Meric-Bernstam F; Kuerer HM; Bedrosian I; Crosby MA; Baumann DP; Ross MI; Feig BW; Krishnamurthy S; Hernandez M; Babiera GV
Institution:	Department of Surgical Oncology, The University of Texas MD Anderson Cancer Center, Houston, TX, USA.
Journal:	Ann Surg Oncol. 2012 Apr;19(4):1137-44. Epub 2011 Oct 7.
Abstract Link:	http://www.medifocus.com/abstracts.php?gid=OC008&ID=21979111

Go to http://www.medifocus.com/links/OC008/0814 for direct online access to the above Abstract Links.

128.

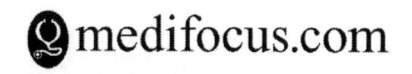

Factors associated with residual disease after initial breast-conserving surgery for ductal carcinoma in situ.

Authors:	Wei S; Kragel CP; Zhang K; Hameed O
Institution:	Department of Pathology, School of Medicine, University of Alabama at Birmingham, Birmingham, AL 35249-7331, USA. swei@uab.edu
Journal:	Hum Pathol. 2012 Jul;43(7):986-93. doi: 10.1016/j.humpath.2011.09.010. Epub 2012 Jan 4.
Abstract Link:	http://www.medifocus.com/abstracts.php?gid=OC008&ID=22221704

129.

Mastectomy and contralateral prophylactic mastectomy rates: an institutional review.

Authors:	Damle S; Teal CB; Lenert JJ; Marshall EC; Pan Q; McSwain AP
Institution:	Department of Surgery, Breast Care Center, The George Washington University, Washington, DC, USA.
Journal:	Ann Surg Oncol. 2011 May;18(5):1356-63. Epub 2010 Dec 2.
Abstract Link:	http://www.medifocus.com/abstracts.php?gid=OC008&ID=21125335

130.

Comparative effectiveness of ductal carcinoma in situ management and the roles of margins and surgeons.

Authors:	Dick AW; Sorbero MS; Ahrendt GM; Hayman JA; Gold HT; Schiffhauer L; Stark A; Griggs JJ
Institution:	The RAND Corporation, Pittsburgh, PA 15213, USA. andrew_dick@rand.org
Journal:	J Natl Cancer Inst. 2011 Jan 19;103(2):92-104. Epub 2011 Jan 3.
Abstract Link:	http://www.medifocus.com/abstracts.php?gid=OC008&ID=21200025

Go to http://www.medifocus.com/links/OC008/0814 for direct online access to the above Abstract Links.

131.

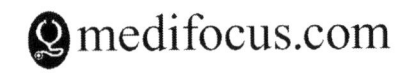

Institutional variation in the surgical treatment of breast cancer: a study of the NCCN.

Authors:	Greenberg CC; Lipsitz SR; Hughes ME; Edge SB; Theriault R; Wilson JL; Carter WB; Blayney DW; Niland J; Weeks JC
Institution:	Center for Outcomes and Policy Research, Department of Medical Oncology, Dana-Farber Cancer Institute, Boston, MA, USA. ccgreenberg@partners.org
Journal:	Ann Surg. 2011 Aug;254(2):339-45.
Abstract Link:	http://www.medifocus.com/abstracts.php?gid=OC008&ID=21725233

132.

Areola and nipple-areola-sparing mastectomy for breast cancer treatment and risk reduction: report of an initial experience in a community hospital setting.

Authors:	Harness JK; Vetter TS; Salibian AH
Institution:	St. Joseph Hospital, The Center for Cancer Treatment and Prevention, Orange, CA, USA. jkharness@aol.com
Journal:	Ann Surg Oncol. 2011 Apr;18(4):917-22. Epub 2010 Oct 7.
Abstract Link:	http://www.medifocus.com/abstracts.php?gid=OC008&ID=21308484

133.

Nipple-sparing mastectomy in 99 patients with a mean follow-up of 5 years.

Authors:	Jensen JA; Orringer JS; Giuliano AE
Institution:	Department of Surgical Oncology, John Wayne Cancer Institute at Saint John's Health Center, Santa Monica, CA, USA.
Journal:	Ann Surg Oncol. 2011 Jun;18(6):1665-70. Epub 2010 Dec 21.
Abstract Link:	http://www.medifocus.com/abstracts.php?gid=OC008&ID=21174155

Go to http://www.medifocus.com/links/OC008/0814 for direct online access to the above Abstract Links.

134.

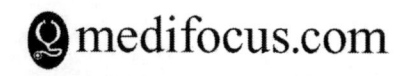

Analyzing the risk of recurrence after mastectomy for DCIS: a new use for the USC/Van Nuys Prognostic Index.

Authors:	Kelley L; Silverstein M; Guerra L
Institution:	Department of Surgical Oncology, University of Southern California, Los Angeles, USA. leah.m.kelley@gmail.com
Journal:	Ann Surg Oncol. 2011 Feb;18(2):459-62. Epub 2010 Sep 22.
Abstract Link:	http://www.medifocus.com/abstracts.php?gid=OC008&ID=20859695

135.

Nomogram for risk of relapse after breast-conserving surgery in ductal carcinoma in situ.

Authors:	Mazouni C; Delaloge S; Rimareix F; Garbay JR
Journal:	J Clin Oncol. 2011 Jan 10;29(2):e44; author reply e45-6. Epub 2010 Dec 6.
Abstract Link:	**ABSTRACT NOT AVAILABLE**

136.

Nipple discharge after nipple-sparing mastectomy: should the areola complex always be removed?

Authors:	Orzalesi L; Aldrovandi S; Calabrese C; Casella D; Brancato B; Cataliotti L
Institution:	Breast Unit, University of Florence, Viale Morgagni 85, Florence, Italy. lorenzo.orzalesi@unifi.it
Journal:	Clin Breast Cancer. 2011 Aug;11(4):270-2. Epub 2011 May 3.
Abstract Link:	http://www.medifocus.com/abstracts.php?gid=OC008&ID=21729659

Go to http://www.medifocus.com/links/OC008/0814 for direct online access to the above Abstract Links.

137.

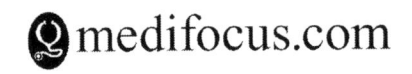

Predictors of local recurrence in a population-based cohort of women with ductal carcinoma in situ treated with breast conserving surgery alone.

Authors:	Wai ES; Lesperance ML; Alexander CS; Truong PT; Moccia P; Culp M; Lindquist J; Olivotto IA
Institution:	Radiation Therapy Program, BC Cancer Agency-Vancouver Island Centre, Victoria, BC, Canada. ewai@bccancer.bc.ca
Journal:	Ann Surg Oncol. 2011 Jan;18(1):119-24. Epub 2010 Jul 20.
Abstract Link:	http://www.medifocus.com/abstracts.php?gid=OC008&ID=20645008

138.

The surgical management of ductal carcinoma in situ.

Authors:	Kumar S; Sacchini V
Institution:	Breast Service, Department of Surgery, Memorial Sloan-Kettering Cancer Center, New York, New York, USA.
Journal:	Breast J. 2010 Sep-Oct;16 Suppl 1:S49-52. doi: 10.1111/j.1524-4741.2010.01005.x.
Abstract Link:	http://www.medifocus.com/abstracts.php?gid=OC008&ID=21050311

139.

Perspectives on margins in DCIS: pathology.

Author:	Lester S
Institution:	Department of Pathology, Brigham and Women's Hospital, Harvard Medical School, Boston, Massachusetts 02115, USA.
Journal:	J Natl Compr Canc Netw. 2010 Oct;8(10):1219-22.
Abstract Link:	http://www.medifocus.com/abstracts.php?gid=OC008&ID=20971844

Go to http://www.medifocus.com/links/OC008/0814 for direct online access to the above Abstract Links.

140.

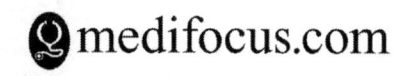

Outcomes evaluation following bilateral breast reconstruction using latissimus dorsi myocutaneous flaps.

Authors:	Losken A; Nicholas CS; Pinell XA; Carlson GW
Institution:	Emory University School of Medicine, Atlanta, GA, USA. alosken@emory.edu <alosken@emory.edu>
Journal:	Ann Plast Surg. 2010 Jul;65(1):17-22.
Abstract Link:	http://www.medifocus.com/abstracts.php?gid=OC008&ID=20548235

141.

Oncological outcome and patient satisfaction with skin-sparing mastectomy and immediate breast reconstruction: a prospective observational study.

Authors:	Reefy S; Patani N; Anderson A; Burgoyne G; Osman H; Mokbel K
Institution:	The London Breast Institute, The Princess Grace Hospital, London, UK.
Journal:	BMC Cancer. 2010 Apr 29;10:171.
Abstract Link:	http://www.medifocus.com/abstracts.php?gid=OC008&ID=20429922

142.

Surgical treatment in Paget's disease of the breast.

Authors:	Siponen E; Hukkinen K; Heikkila P; Joensuu H; Leidenius M
Institution:	Helsinki University Central Hospital, Finland. elina.siponen@elisanet.fi
Journal:	Am J Surg. 2010 Aug;200(2):241-6.
Abstract Link:	http://www.medifocus.com/abstracts.php?gid=OC008&ID=20678619

Go to http://www.medifocus.com/links/OC008/0814 for direct online access to the above Abstract Links.

143.

Trends in contralateral prophylactic mastectomy for unilateral cancer: a report from the National Cancer Data Base, 1998-2007.

Authors:	Yao K; Stewart AK; Winchester DJ; Winchester DP
Institution:	Department of Surgery, University of Chicago, Pritzker School of Medicine, NorthShore University Health System, Evanston Hospital, Evanston, IL, USA. kyao@northshore.org
Journal:	Ann Surg Oncol. 2010 Oct;17(10):2554-62. Epub 2010 May 12.
Abstract Link:	http://www.medifocus.com/abstracts.php?gid=OC008&ID=20461470

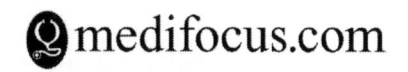

Clinical Trials Articles

144.

Anastrozole for prevention of breast cancer in high-risk postmenopausal women (IBIS-II): an international, double-blind, randomised placebo-controlled trial.

Authors:	Cuzick J; Sestak I; Forbes JF; Dowsett M; Knox J; Cawthorn S; Saunders C; Roche N; Mansel RE; von Minckwitz G; Bonanni B; Palva T; Howell A
Institution:	Array Italy.; Pirkanmaa Cancer Society, Tampere, Finland.; Genesis Breast Cancer Prevention Centre, Manchester, UK.
Journal:	Lancet. 2014 Mar 22;383(9922):1041-8. doi: 10.1016/S0140-6736(13)62292-8. Epub 2013 Dec 12.
Abstract Link:	http://www.medifocus.com/abstracts.php?gid=OC008&ID=24333009

145.

Two different hypofractionated breast radiotherapy schedules for 113 patients with ductal carcinoma in situ: preliminary results.

Authors:	Guenzi M; Giannelli F; Bosetti D; Blandino G; Milanese ML; Pupillo F; Corvo R; Fozza A
Institution:	Oncologia Radioterapica, IRCCS A.O.U. San Martino-IST-Istituto Nazionale per la Ricerca, sul Cancro, Largo R. Benzi, 10, 16132 Genoa, Italy. ale.fozza@libero.it
Journal:	Anticancer Res. 2013 Aug;33(8):3503-7.
Abstract Link:	http://www.medifocus.com/abstracts.php?gid=OC008&ID=23898126

Go to http://www.medifocus.com/links/OC008/0814 for direct online access to the above Abstract Links.

146.

Hypofractionated radiation therapy for breast ductal carcinoma in situ.

Authors:	Hathout L; Hijal T; Theberge V; Fortin B; Vulpe H; Hogue JC; Lambert C; Bahig H; Provencher L; Vavassis P; Yassa M
Institution:	Department of Radiation Oncology, Hopital Maisonneuve-Rosemont, Centre affilie a l'Universite de Montreal, Montreal, Quebec, Canada.
Journal:	Int J Radiat Oncol Biol Phys. 2013 Dec 1;87(5):1058-63. doi: 10.1016/j.ijrobp.2013.08.026. Epub 2013 Oct 8.
Abstract Link:	http://www.medifocus.com/abstracts.php?gid=OC008&ID=24113057

147.

The clinical significance of breast MRI in the management of ductal carcinoma in situ diagnosed on needle biopsy.

Authors:	Miyashita M; Amano G; Ishida T; Tamaki K; Uchimura F; Ono T; Yajima M; Kuriya Y; Ohuchi N
Institution:	Department of Surgery and Breast Surgery, Nihonkai General Hospital, 30 Akiho-cho, Sakata 998-8501, Japan. atihsayim8m8@med.tohoku.ac.jp
Journal:	Jpn J Clin Oncol. 2013 Jun;43(6):654-63. doi: 10.1093/jjco/hyt055. Epub 2013 Apr 16.
Abstract Link:	http://www.medifocus.com/abstracts.php?gid=OC008&ID=23592884

148.

Five year outcome of 145 patients with ductal carcinoma in situ (DCIS) after accelerated breast radiotherapy.

Authors:	Ciervide R; Dhage S; Guth A; Shapiro RL; Axelrod DM; Roses DF; Formenti SC
Institution:	Department of Radiation Oncology, New York University School of Medicine, NYU Langone Medical Center, New York, New York, USA.
Journal:	Int J Radiat Oncol Biol Phys. 2012 Jun 1;83(2):e159-64.
Abstract Link:	http://www.medifocus.com/abstracts.php?gid=OC008&ID=22579378

Go to http://www.medifocus.com/links/OC008/0814 for direct online access to the above Abstract Links.

149.

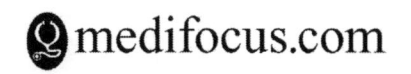

Ten-year risk of diagnostic mammograms and invasive breast procedures after breast-conserving surgery for DCIS.

Authors:	Nekhlyudov L; Habel LA; Achacoso N; Jung I; Haque R; Collins LC; Schnitt SJ; Quesenberry CP Jr; Fletcher SW
Institution:	Department of Population Medicine, Harvard Medical School and Harvard Pilgrim Health Care Institute, 133 Brookline Ave, 6th Floor, Boston, MA 02215, USA. larissa_nekhlyudov@harvardpilgrim.org
Journal:	J Natl Cancer Inst. 2012 Apr 18;104(8):614-21. Epub 2012 Apr 5.
Abstract Link:	http://www.medifocus.com/abstracts.php?gid=OC008&ID=22491230

150.

Multi-institutional experience of ductal carcinoma in situ in black vs white patients treated with breast-conserving surgery and whole breast radiation therapy.

Authors:	Nelson C; Bai H; Neboori H; Takita C; Motwani S; Wright JL; Hobeika G; Haffty BG; Jones T; Goyal S; Moran MS
Institution:	Robert Wood Johnson Medical School, New Brunswick, New Jersey, USA.
Journal:	Int J Radiat Oncol Biol Phys. 2012 Nov 1;84(3):e279-83. doi: 10.1016/j.ijrobp.2012.03.068. Epub 2012 Jun 5.
Abstract Link:	http://www.medifocus.com/abstracts.php?gid=OC008&ID=22672752

151.

Effect of tamoxifen and radiotherapy in women with locally excised ductal carcinoma in situ: long-term results from the UK/ANZ DCIS trial.

Authors:	Cuzick J; Sestak I; Pinder SE; Ellis IO; Forsyth S; Bundred NJ; Forbes JF; Bishop H; Fentiman IS; George WD
Institution:	Cancer Research UK, Centre for Epidemiology, Mathematics, and Statistics, Wolfson Institute of Preventive Medicine, Queen Mary School of Medicine and Dentistry, University of London, London, UK. j.cuzick@qmul.ac.uk
Journal:	Lancet Oncol. 2011 Jan;12(1):21-9. Epub 2010 Dec 7.
Abstract Link:	http://www.medifocus.com/abstracts.php?gid=OC008&ID=21145284

Go to http://www.medifocus.com/links/OC008/0814 for direct online access to the above Abstract Links.

152.

Long-term outcomes of invasive ipsilateral breast tumor recurrences after lumpectomy in NSABP B-17 and B-24 randomized clinical trials for DCIS.

Authors:	Wapnir IL; Dignam JJ; Fisher B; Mamounas EP; Anderson SJ; Julian TB; Land SR; Margolese RG; Swain SM; Costantino JP; Wolmark N
Institution:	Department of Surgery; 300 Pasteur Dr H3625, Stanford University School of Medicine, Stanford, CA 94305-5655. wapnir@stanford.edu.
Journal:	J Natl Cancer Inst. 2011 Mar 16;103(6):478-88. Epub 2011 Mar 11.
Abstract Link:	http://www.medifocus.com/abstracts.php?gid=OC008&ID=21398619

153.

Five-year outcome of patients classified in the "unsuitable" category using the American Society of Therapeutic Radiology and Oncology (ASTRO) Consensus Panel guidelines for the application of accelerated partial breast irradiation: an analysis of patients treated on the American Society of Breast Surgeons MammoSite(R) Registry trial.

Authors:	Beitsch P; Vicini F; Keisch M; Haffty B; Shaitelman S; Lyden M
Institution:	Surgery, Dallas Breast Center, Dallas, TX, USA. Beitsch@aol.com
Journal:	Ann Surg Oncol. 2010 Oct;17 Suppl 3:219-25. Epub 2010 Sep 19.
Abstract Link:	http://www.medifocus.com/abstracts.php?gid=OC008&ID=20853036

154.

Lesion size is a major determinant of the mammographic features of ductal carcinoma in situ: findings from the Sloane project.

Authors:	Evans A; Clements K; Maxwell A; Bishop H; Hanby A; Lawrence G; Pinder SE
Institution:	Ninewells Hospital and Medical School, Dundee, Scotland, UK. a.z.evans@dundee.ac.uk
Journal:	Clin Radiol. 2010 Mar;65(3):181-4. Epub 2010 Jan 18.
Abstract Link:	http://www.medifocus.com/abstracts.php?gid=OC008&ID=20152272

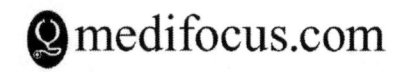

Radiation Therapy Articles

155.

Role of radiotherapy boost in women with ductal carcinoma in situ: a single-center experience in a series of 389 patients.

Authors:	Meattini I; Livi L; Franceschini D; Saieva C; Meacci F; Marrazzo L; Bendinelli B; Scotti V; De Luca Cardillo C; Nori J; Sanchez L; Orzalesi L; Bonomo P; Greto D; Bucciolini M; Bianchi S; Biti G
Institution:	Radiotherapy Unit, University of Florence, FLargo G. A. Brambilla 3, lorence, Italy. icro.meattini@unifi.it
Journal:	Eur J Surg Oncol. 2013 Jun;39(6):613-8. doi: 10.1016/j.ejso.2013.03.002. Epub 2013 Mar 20.
Abstract Link:	http://www.medifocus.com/abstracts.php?gid=OC008&ID=23523088

156.

Impact of boost radiation in the treatment of ductal carcinoma in situ: a population-based analysis.

Authors:	Rakovitch E; Narod SA; Nofech-Moses S; Hanna W; Thiruchelvam D; Saskin R; Taylor C; Tuck A; Youngson B; Miller N; Done SJ; Sengupta S; Elavathil L; Jani PA; Bonin M; Metcalfe S; Paszat L
Institution:	Sunnybrook Health Sciences Centre, 2075 Bayview Avenue, Toronto, Ontario, Canada. Eileen.rakovitch@sunnybrook.ca
Journal:	Int J Radiat Oncol Biol Phys. 2013 Jul 1;86(3):491-7. doi: 10.1016/j.ijrobp.2013.02.031.
Abstract Link:	http://www.medifocus.com/abstracts.php?gid=OC008&ID=23708085

Go to http://www.medifocus.com/links/OC008/0814 for direct online access to the above Abstract Links.

157.

Tumor bed control with balloon-based accelerated partial breast irradiation: incidence of true recurrences versus elsewhere failures in the American Society of Breast Surgery MammoSite((R)) Registry Trial.

Authors:	Beitsch PD; Wilkinson JB; Vicini FA; Haffty B; Fine R; Whitworth P; Kuerer H; Zannis V; Lyden M
Institution:	Department of Surgery, Dallas Breast Center, Dallas, TX, USA. beitsch@aol.com
Journal:	Ann Surg Oncol. 2012 Oct;19(10):3165-70. doi: 10.1245/s10434-012-2489-x. Epub 2012 Jul 27.
Abstract Link:	http://www.medifocus.com/abstracts.php?gid=OC008&ID=22836556

158.

Cost comparison of radiation treatment options after lumpectomy for breast cancer.

Authors:	Greenup RA; Camp MS; Taghian AG; Buckley J; Coopey SB; Gadd M; Hughes K; Specht M; Smith BL
Institution:	Division of Surgical Oncology, Massachusetts General Hospital, Boston, MA, USA. rgreenup13@gmail.com
Journal:	Ann Surg Oncol. 2012 Oct;19(10):3275-81. doi: 10.1245/s10434-012-2546-5. Epub 2012 Aug 1.
Abstract Link:	http://www.medifocus.com/abstracts.php?gid=OC008&ID=22851048

159.

Radiation therapy for ductal carcinoma in situ: a decision analysis.

Authors:	Punglia RS; Burstein HJ; Weeks JC
Institution:	Department of Radiation Oncology, Dana-Farber Cancer Institute/Brigham and Women's Hospital, Harvard Medical School, Boston, Massachusetts 02115, USA. rpunglia@lroc.harvard.edu
Journal:	Cancer. 2012 Feb 1;118(3):603-11. doi: 10.1002/cncr.26293. Epub 2011 Jun 30.
Abstract Link:	http://www.medifocus.com/abstracts.php?gid=OC008&ID=21720992

Go to http://www.medifocus.com/links/OC008/0814 for direct online access to the above Abstract Links.

160.

Skin toxicity and cosmesis after hypofractionated whole breast irradiation for early breast cancer.

Authors:	Saksornchai K; Rojpornpradit P; Shotelersak K; Lertbutsayanukul C; Chakkabat C; Raiyawa T
Institution:	Division of Therapeutic Radiology and Oncology, Department of Radiology, Faculty of Medicine, Chulalongkorn University, Bangkok, Thailand.
Journal:	J Med Assoc Thai. 2012 Feb;95(2):229-40.
Abstract Link:	http://www.medifocus.com/abstracts.php?gid=OC008&ID=22435254

161.

Ductal carcinoma in situ--the influence of the radiotherapy boost on local control.

Authors:	Wong P; Lambert C; Agnihotram RV; David M; Duclos M; Freeman CR
Institution:	Division of Radiation Oncology, McGill University Health Centre, Montreal, QC, Canada.
Journal:	Int J Radiat Oncol Biol Phys. 2012 Feb 1;82(2):e153-8. Epub 2011 Jun 12.
Abstract Link:	http://www.medifocus.com/abstracts.php?gid=OC008&ID=21664063

162.

Outcomes in women treated with MammoSite brachytherapy or whole breast irradiation stratified by ASTRO Accelerated Partial Breast Irradiation Consensus Statement Groups.

Authors:	Zauls AJ; Watkins JM; Wahlquist AE; Brackett NC 3rd; Aguero EG; Baker MK; Jenrette JM; Garrett-Mayer E; Harper JL
Institution:	Department of Radiation Oncology, Medical University of South Carolina, Charleston, SC 29425, USA. zauls@musc.edu
Journal:	Int J Radiat Oncol Biol Phys. 2012 Jan 1;82(1):21-9. Epub 2010 Oct 15.
Abstract Link:	http://www.medifocus.com/abstracts.php?gid=OC008&ID=20951508

Go to http://www.medifocus.com/links/OC008/0814 for direct online access to the above Abstract Links.

163.

Accelerated partial breast irradiation for pure ductal carcinoma in situ.

Authors:	Park SS; Grills IS; Chen PY; Kestin LL; Ghilezan MI; Wallace M; Martinez AM; Vicini FA
Institution:	Department of Radiation Oncology, William Beaumont Hospital, Royal Oak, MI 48073, USA.
Journal:	Int J Radiat Oncol Biol Phys. 2011 Oct 1;81(2):403-8. Epub 2010 Aug 26.
Abstract Link:	http://www.medifocus.com/abstracts.php?gid=OC008&ID=20800374

164.

Ductal carcinoma in situ of the breast treated with accelerated partial breast irradiation using balloon-based brachytherapy.

Authors:	Israel PZ; Vicini F; Robbins AB; Shroff P; McLaughlin M; Grier K; Lyden M
Institution:	The Breast Center, Marietta, GA, USA. pzisrael@aol.com
Journal:	Ann Surg Oncol. 2010 Nov;17(11):2940-4. Epub 2010 May 5.
Abstract Link:	http://www.medifocus.com/abstracts.php?gid=OC008&ID=20443148

165.

The influence of margin width and volume of disease near margin on benefit of radiation therapy for women with DCIS treated with breast-conserving therapy.

Authors:	Rudloff U; Brogi E; Reiner AS; Goldberg JI; Brockway JP; Wynveen CA; McCormick B; Patil S; Van Zee KJ
Institution:	Breast Service, Department of Surgery, Memorial Sloan-Kettering Cancer Center, New York, NY 10065, USA.
Journal:	Ann Surg. 2010 Apr;251(4):583-91.
Abstract Link:	http://www.medifocus.com/abstracts.php?gid=OC008&ID=20224381

Go to http://www.medifocus.com/links/OC008/0814 for direct online access to the above Abstract Links.

166.

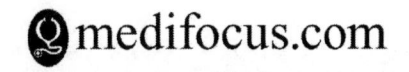

Local control with conventional and hypofractionated adjuvant radiotherapy after breast-conserving surgery for ductal carcinoma in-situ.

Authors:	Williamson D; Dinniwell R; Fung S; Pintilie M; Done SJ; Fyles AW
Institution:	Radiation Medicine Program, Princess Margaret Hospital, Department of Radiation Oncology, University of Toronto, Canada M5G2M9.
Journal:	Radiother Oncol. 2010 Jun;95(3):317-20. Epub 2010 Apr 17.
Abstract Link:	http://www.medifocus.com/abstracts.php?gid=OC008&ID=20400190

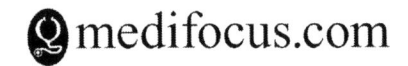

NOTES

Use this page for taking notes as you review your Guidebook

4 - Centers of Research

This section of your *MediFocus Guidebook* is a unique directory of doctors, researchers, medical centers, and research institutions with specialized research interest, and in many cases, clinical expertise in the management of this specific medical condition. The *Centers of Research* directory is a valuable resource for quickly identifying and locating leading medical authorities and medical institutions within the United States and other countries that are considered to be at the forefront in clinical research and treatment of this disorder.

Use the *Centers of Research* directory to contact, consult, or network with leading experts in the field and to locate a hospital or medical center that can help you.

The following information is provided in the *Centers of Research* directory:

- **Geographic Location**

    - United States: the information is divided by individual states listed in alphabetical order. Not all states may be included.

    - Other Countries: information is presented for select countries worldwide listed in alphabetical order. Not all countries may be included.

- **Names of Authors**

    - Select names of individual authors (doctors, researchers, or other health-care professionals) with specialized research interest, and in many cases, clinical expertise in the management of this specific medical condition, who have recently published articles in leading medical journals about the condition.

    - E-mail addresses for individual authors, if listed on their specific publications, is also provided.

- **Institutional Affiliations**

    - Next to each individual author's name is their **institutional affiliation** (hospital, medical center, or research institution) where the study was conducted as listed in their publication(s).

- In many cases, information about the specific **department** within the medical institution where the individual author was located at the time the study was conducted is also provided.

Centers of Research

United States

AL - Alabama

Name of Author	Institutional Affiliation
Hameed O	Department of Pathology, School of Medicine, University of Alabama at Birmingham, Birmingham, AL 35249-7331, USA. swei@uab.edu
Wei S	Department of Pathology, School of Medicine, University of Alabama at Birmingham, Birmingham, AL 35249-7331, USA. swei@uab.edu

AZ - Arizona

Name of Author	Institutional Affiliation
Gray RJ	Section of Surgical Oncology, Department of Surgery, Mayo Clinic Hospital, Mayo Clinic, Phoenix, AZ, USA.
McGhan LJ	Section of Surgical Oncology, Department of Surgery, Mayo Clinic Hospital, Mayo Clinic, Phoenix, AZ, USA.

CA - California

Name of Author	Institutional Affiliation
Ganz PA	Division of Cancer Prevention and Control Research, Jonsson Comprehensive Cancer Center, 650 Charles Young Dr South, Rm A2-125 CHS, Los Angeles, CA 90095-6900, USA. pganz@ucla.edu
Giuliano AE	Division of Plastic Surgery, Geffen School of Medicine at U.C.L.A., Los Angeles, CA, USA. Dr.J.Jensen@gmail.com
Guerra L	Department of Surgical Oncology, University of Southern California, Los Angeles, USA. leah.m.kelley@gmail.com

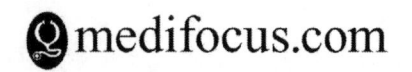

Harness JK	St. Joseph Hospital, The Center for Cancer Treatment and Prevention, Orange, CA, USA. jkharness@aol.com
Hwang ES	Department of Surgery and Helen Diller Family Comprehensive Cancer Center, University of California, San Francisco, San Francisco, CA 94115, USA. shelley.hwang@ucsfmedctr.org
Jensen JA	Division of Plastic Surgery, Geffen School of Medicine at U.C.L.A., Los Angeles, CA, USA. Dr.J.Jensen@gmail.com
Kelley L	Department of Surgical Oncology, University of Southern California, Los Angeles, USA. leah.m.kelley@gmail.com
Kerlikowske K	University of California, San Francisco, CA 94121, USA. karla.kerlikowkse@ucsf.edu
Lagios MD	Breast Program, Hoag Memorial Hospital Presbyterian, Newport Beach, CA , USA. melsilver9@gmail.com
Love SM	Department of Surgery, St Joseph Health, Eureka, CA, USA.
Mahoney ME	Department of Surgery, St Joseph Health, Eureka, CA, USA.
Martinez SR	Department of Surgery, Division of Surgical Oncology, University of California Davis, Sacramento, California, USA.
Salibian AH	St. Joseph Hospital, The Center for Cancer Treatment and Prevention, Orange, CA, USA. jkharness@aol.com
Schmale I	Division of Breast and Soft Tissue Surgery, Department of Surgery, Keck School of Medicine, University of Southern California, Los Angeles, California, USA.
Sener SF	Division of Breast and Soft Tissue Surgery, Department of Surgery, Keck School of Medicine, University of Southern California, Los Angeles, California, USA.
Shah DR	Department of Surgery, Division of Surgical Oncology, University of California Davis, Sacramento, California, USA.
Silverstein MJ	Breast Program, Hoag Memorial Hospital Presbyterian, Newport Beach, CA , USA. melsilver9@gmail.com

Tlsty TD	University of California, San Francisco, CA 94121, USA. karla.kerlikowkse@ucsf.edu
Wapnir IL	Department of Surgery; 300 Pasteur Dr H3625, Stanford University School of Medicine, Stanford, CA 94305-5655. wapnir@stanford.edu.
Wolmark N	Department of Surgery; 300 Pasteur Dr H3625, Stanford University School of Medicine, Stanford, CA 94305-5655. wapnir@stanford.edu.

CT - Connecticut

Name of Author	Institutional Affiliation
Chagpar AB	Department of Surgery, Yale University School of Medicine, New Haven, Connecticut, USA.
Sue GR	Department of Surgery, Yale University School of Medicine, New Haven, Connecticut, USA.

DC - Washington D.C.

Name of Author	Institutional Affiliation
Damle S	Department of Surgery, Breast Care Center, The George Washington University, Washington, DC, USA.
Eng-Wong J	Department of Internal Medicine, Division of Oncology, Lombardi Cancer Center, Georgetown University, Washington, DC, USA.
McSwain AP	Department of Surgery, Breast Care Center, The George Washington University, Washington, DC, USA.
Swain SM	Department of Internal Medicine, Division of Oncology, Lombardi Cancer Center, Georgetown University, Washington, DC, USA.

FL - Florida

Name of Author	Institutional Affiliation
Allegra CJ	University of Florida Shands Cancer Center, Department of Medicine, University of Florida, Gainesville, FL 32610, USA. carmen.allegra@medicine.ufl.edu
Masood S	Department of Pathology, University of Florida College of Medicine, Jacksonville, FL, USA. shahla.masood@jax.ufl.edu
Zon R	University of Florida Shands Cancer Center, Department of Medicine, University of Florida, Gainesville, FL 32610, USA. carmen.allegra@medicine.ufl.edu

GA - Georgia

Name of Author	Institutional Affiliation
Carlson GW	Emory University School of Medicine, Atlanta, GA, USA. alosken@emory.edu <alosken@emory.edu>
D'Orsi CJ	Department of Radiology, Breast Imaging Center, Emory University Hospital, WCI Bldg, 1365-C Clifton Rd, Ste C1104, Atlanta, GA 30322, USA. carl_dorsi@emoryhealthcare.org
Israel PZ	The Breast Center, Marietta, GA, USA. pzisrael@aol.com
Losken A	Emory University School of Medicine, Atlanta, GA, USA. alosken@emory.edu <alosken@emory.edu>
Lyden M	The Breast Center, Marietta, GA, USA. pzisrael@aol.com

IL - Illinois

Name of Author	Institutional Affiliation
Jeruss JS	Department of Surgery, Northwestern University Feinberg School of Medicine, Chicago, IL, USA. jjeruss@nmh.org
Kantor O	University of Chicago, Pritzker School of Medicine, Chicago, Illinois.

Keisch M	Department of Surgery, Northwestern University Feinberg School of Medicine, Chicago, IL, USA. jjeruss@nmh.org
Melstrom LG	Department of Surgery, Northwestern University, Chicago, IL, USA.
Siziopikou KP	Breast Pathology Service, Northwestern University Feinberg School of Medicine, Chicago, Illinois, USA. p-siziopikou@northwestern.edu
Winchester DJ	Department of Surgery, Northwestern University, Chicago, IL, USA.
Winchester DP	Department of Surgery, University of Chicago, Pritzker School of Medicine, NorthShore University Health System, Evanston Hospital, Evanston, IL, USA. kyao@northshore.org
Yao K	Department of Surgery, University of Chicago, Pritzker School of Medicine, NorthShore University Health System, Evanston Hospital, Evanston, IL, USA. kyao@northshore.org

IN - Indiana

Name of Author	Institutional Affiliation
Luo J	Department of Epidemiology and Biostatistics, School of Public Health-Bloomington, Indiana University, Bloomington, IN, USA. juhluo@indiana.edu
Margolis KL	Department of Epidemiology and Biostatistics, School of Public Health-Bloomington, Indiana University, Bloomington, IN, USA. juhluo@indiana.edu

KS - Kansas

Name of Author	Institutional Affiliation
Fan F	Department of Pathology and Laboratory Medicine, University of Kansas Medical Center, Kansas City, KS 66160, USA.
Shatat L	Department of Pathology and Laboratory Medicine, University of Kansas Medical Center, Kansas City, KS 66160, USA.

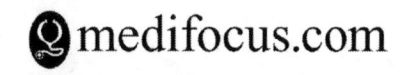

MA - Massachussetts

Name of Author	Institutional Affiliation
Arvold ND	Harvard Radiation Oncology Program, Harvard Medical School, Boston, Massachusetts, USA. narvold@partners.org
Bellon JR	Harvard Radiation Oncology Program, Boston, MA 02115, USA.
Bober SL	Dana-Farber Cancer Institute, Brigham and Women's Hospital and Harvard Medical School, Boston, MA, USA. Sharon_Bober@dfci.harvard.edu
Bombonati A	Department of Pathology, Harvard Medical School, Molecular Pathology Research Unit, Massachusetts General Hospital, Boston, MA, USA.
Brock JE	Harvard Radiation Oncology Program, Boston, MA, USA.
Childs SK	Harvard Radiation Oncology Program, Boston, MA 02115, USA.
Fletcher SW	Department of Population Medicine, Harvard Medical School and Harvard Pilgrim Health Care Institute, 133 Brookline Ave, 6th Floor, Boston, MA 02215, USA. larissa_nekhlyudov@harvardpilgrim.org
Greenberg CC	Center for Outcomes and Policy Research, Department of Medical Oncology, Dana-Farber Cancer Institute, Boston, MA, USA. ccgreenberg@partners.org
Greenup RA	Division of Surgical Oncology, Massachusetts General Hospital, Boston, MA, USA. rgreenup13@gmail.com
Halasz LM	Harvard Radiation Oncology Program, Boston, MA, USA.
Hassett MJ	Harvard Radiation Oncology Program, Harvard Medical School, Boston, Massachusetts, USA. narvold@partners.org
Lester S	Department of Pathology, Brigham and Women's Hospital, Harvard Medical School, Boston, Massachusetts 02115, USA.
Nekhlyudov L	Department of Population Medicine, Harvard Medical School and Harvard Pilgrim Health Care Institute, 133 Brookline Ave, 6th Floor, Boston, MA 02215, USA. larissa_nekhlyudov@harvardpilgrim.org

Partridge A	Dana-Farber Cancer Institute, Brigham and Women's Hospital and Harvard Medical School, Boston, MA, USA. Sharon_Bober@dfci.harvard.edu
Polyak K	Department of Medical Oncology, Dana-Farber Cancer Institute, 44 Binney St D740C, Boston, MA 02115, USA. kornelia_polyak@dfci.harvard.edu
Punglia RS	Center for Health Decision Science, Department of Health Policy and Management, Harvard School of Public Health, Boston, MA 02115, USA. dsoetema@hsph.harvard.edu
Schnitt SJ	Department of Pathology, Beth Israel Deaconess Medical Center, 330 Brookline Ave, Boston, MA 02215, USA. sschnitt@bidmc.harvard.edu
Sgroi DC	Department of Pathology, Harvard Medical School, Molecular Pathology Research Unit, Massachusetts General Hospital, Boston, MA, USA.
Smith BL	Division of Surgical Oncology, Massachusetts General Hospital, Boston, MA, USA. rgreenup13@gmail.com
Soeteman DI	Center for Health Decision Science, Department of Health Policy and Management, Harvard School of Public Health, Boston, MA 02115, USA. dsoetema@hsph.harvard.edu
Weeks JC	Department of Radiation Oncology, Dana-Farber Cancer Institute/Brigham and Women's Hospital, Harvard Medical School, Boston, Massachusetts 02115, USA. rpunglia@lroc.harvard.edu

MD - Maryland

Name of Author	Institutional Affiliation
Jansen SA	Mouse Cancer Genetics Program, National Cancer Institute, Frederick, MD, USA. jansena@mail.nih.gov
Stevens JL	National Cancer Institute, CTEP, Bethesda, MD, USA.
Zujewski JA	National Cancer Institute, CTEP, Bethesda, MD, USA.

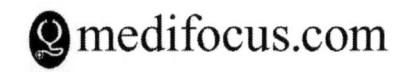

MI - Michigan

Name of Author	Institutional Affiliation
Nassar Warzecha H	Department of Pathology, Wayne State University, Detroit, MI 48201, USA. bsharafa@med.wayne.edu
Newman LA	Department of Surgery, Breast Care Center, University of Michigan Comprehensive Cancer Center, 1500 East Medical Center Dr, 3308 Cancer Center, Ann Arbor, MI 48109-0932, USA. lanewman@umich.edu
Park SS	Department of Radiation Oncology, William Beaumont Hospital, Royal Oak, MI 48073, USA.
Sharaf Aldeen B	Department of Pathology, Wayne State University, Detroit, MI 48201, USA. bsharafa@med.wayne.edu
Vicini FA	Department of Radiation Oncology, William Beaumont Hospital, Royal Oak, MI 48073, USA.

MN - Minnesota

Name of Author	Institutional Affiliation
Ansari B	Department of Surgery, Mayo Clinic, Rochester, MN, USA.
Kane RL	Division of Health Policy and Management, University of Minnesota School of Public Health, A365 Mayo (MMC 729), Minneapolis, MN 55455, USA. virni001@umn.edu
Morton MJ	Department of Surgery, Mayo Clinic, Rochester, MN, USA.
Shamliyan T	Division of Health Policy and Management, University of Minnesota School of Public Health, D330-5 Mayo (MMC 729), 420 Delaware St SE, Minneapolis, MN 55455, USA. shaml005@umn.edu
Tuttle TM	Department of Surgery, University of Minnesota, 420 Delaware St SE, Minneapolis, MN 55455, USA. tuttl006@umn.edu
Virnig BA	Division of Health Policy and Management, University of Minnesota School of Public Health, 420 Delaware St S.E., MMC 729, Minneapolis, MN 55455, USA. wang1018@umn.edu

Wang SY	Division of Health Policy and Management, University of Minnesota School of Public Health, 420 Delaware St S.E., MMC 729, Minneapolis, MN 55455, USA. wang1018@umn.edu
Wilt TJ	Division of Health Policy and Management, University of Minnesota School of Public Health, D351 Mayo (MMC 729), 420 Delaware St SE, Minneapolis, MN 55455, USA. kanex001@umn.edu

MO - Missouri

Name of Author	Institutional Affiliation
Al Mushawah F	Department of Surgery, Washington University School of Medicine, St. Louis, Missouri 63110, USA.
Allred DC	National Surgical Adjuvant Breast and Bowel Project, Washington University School of Medicine, Department of Pathology and Immunology, 660 Euclid Campus Box 8118, St Louis, MO 63110, USA. dcallred@path.wustl.edu
Bunting PW	Department of Surgery, Washington University School of Medicine, St. Louis, Missouri.
Margenthaler JA	Department of Surgery, Washington University School of Medicine, St. Louis, Missouri.
Wolmark N	National Surgical Adjuvant Breast and Bowel Project, Washington University School of Medicine, Department of Pathology and Immunology, 660 Euclid Campus Box 8118, St Louis, MO 63110, USA. dcallred@path.wustl.edu

NH - New Hampshire

Name of Author	Institutional Affiliation
Davis KL	Department of Surgery, Dartmouth Hitchcock Medical Center, Lebanon, NH, USA.
Rosenkranz K	Department of Surgery, Dartmouth Hitchcock Medical Center, Lebanon, NH, USA.

NJ - New Jersey

Name of Author	Institutional Affiliation
Moran MS	The Cancer Institute of New Jersey, University of Medicine and Dentistry, New Jersey-Robert Wood Johnson Medical School, New Brunswick, NJ, USA.
Nelson C	Robert Wood Johnson Medical School, New Brunswick, New Jersey, USA.
Parikh RR	The Cancer Institute of New Jersey, University of Medicine and Dentistry, New Jersey-Robert Wood Johnson Medical School, New Brunswick, NJ, USA.

NY - New York

Name of Author	Institutional Affiliation
Boolbol SK	Department of Surgery, Beth Israel Medical Center, New York, NY, USA.
Ciervide R	Department of Radiation Oncology, New York University School of Medicine, NYU Langone Medical Center, New York, New York, USA.
Formenti SC	Department of Radiation Oncology, New York University School of Medicine, NYU Langone Medical Center, New York, New York, USA.
Guth AA	Department of Radiology, New York University School of Medicine, United States.
Ho A	Department of Radiation Oncology, Memorial Sloan-Kettering Cancer Center, 1275 York Avenue, New York, NY, USA. hoa1234@mskcc.org
Ho AY	Department of Radiation Oncology, Memorial Sloan-Kettering Cancer Center, 1275 York Avenue, New York, NY 10065, USA.
Keto JL	Department of Surgery, Beth Israel Medical Center, New York, NY, USA.
Kumar S	Breast Service, Department of Surgery, Memorial Sloan-Kettering Cancer Center, New York, New York, USA.

Lewis JL	St. Luke's-Roosevelt Hospital Center, New York, NY, USA. janalew@gmail.com
McCormick B	Department of Radiation Oncology, Memorial Sloan-Kettering Cancer Center, 1275 York Avenue, New York, NY, USA. hoa1234@mskcc.org
Rudloff U	Breast Service, Department of Surgery, Memorial Sloan-Kettering Cancer Center, New York, NY 10065, USA.
Sacchini V	Breast Service, Department of Surgery, Memorial Sloan-Kettering Cancer Center, New York, New York, USA.
Tartter PI	St. Luke's-Roosevelt Hospital Center, New York, NY, USA. janalew@gmail.com
Van Zee KJ	Breast Service, Department of Surgery, Memorial Sloan-Kettering Cancer Center, New York, NY 10065, USA.
Vieira CC	Department of Radiology, New York University School of Medicine, United States.
Yang TJ	Department of Radiation Oncology, Memorial Sloan-Kettering Cancer Center, 1275 York Avenue, New York, NY 10065, USA.

OH - Ohio

Name of Author	Institutional Affiliation
Emmons KM	the Ohio State University College of Public Health, Columbus, Ohio, USA. jdemoor@cph.osu.edu
Gunia SR	Affinity Medical Center, Massillon, OH, USA.
Mamounas EP	Affinity Medical Center, Massillon, OH, USA.
de Moor JS	the Ohio State University College of Public Health, Columbus, Ohio, USA. jdemoor@cph.osu.edu

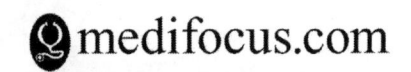

OR - Oregon

Name of Author	Institutional Affiliation
Goddard KA	The Center for Health Research, Kaiser Permanente Northwest, Portland, OR, USA. katrina.ab.goddard@kpchr.org
Wax C	The Center for Health Research, Kaiser Permanente Northwest, Portland, OR, USA. katrina.ab.goddard@kpchr.org

PA - Pennsylvania

Name of Author	Institutional Affiliation
Bleicher RJ	Department of Surgical Oncology, Fox Chase Cancer Center, 333 Cottman Avenue, Room C-308, Philadelphia, PA 19111, USA. richard.bleicher@fccc.edu
Dick AW	The RAND Corporation, Pittsburgh, PA 15213, USA. andrew_dick@rand.org
Freedman GM	Perelman School of Medicine of the University of Pennsylvania, Philadelphia, PA 19104, USA. gary.freedman@uphs.upenn.edu
Griggs JJ	The RAND Corporation, Pittsburgh, PA 15213, USA. andrew_dick@rand.org
Harada S	Department of Pathology and Laboratory Medicine, The University of Pennsylvania, Philadelphia, Pennsylvania, USA.
Holmes P	Department of Pathology, Anatomy, and Cell Biology, Thomas Jefferson University Hospital, Philadelphia, Pennsylvania, USA.
Julian TB	Department of Human Oncology, Allegheny General Hospital, Pittsburgh, PA 15212, USA.
Palazzo JP	Department of Pathology, Anatomy, and Cell Biology, Thomas Jefferson University Hospital, Philadelphia, Pennsylvania, USA.

Shapiro-Wright HM	Department of Human Oncology, Allegheny General Hospital, Pittsburgh, PA 15212, USA.
Solin LJ	Department of Radiation Oncology, Albert Einstein Medical Center, 5501 Old York Rd, Philadelphia, PA 19141, USA. solin@einstein.edu
Zhang PJ	Department of Pathology and Laboratory Medicine, The University of Pennsylvania, Philadelphia, Pennsylvania, USA.

RI - Rhode Island

Name of Author	Institutional Affiliation
Tejada-Berges T	The Warren Alpert School of Medicine of Brown University, Department of Obstetrics and Gynecology, Program in Women's Oncology, Women and Infants' Hospital, Providence, Rhode Island, USA. ttejadaberges@wihri.org

SC - South Carolina

Name of Author	Institutional Affiliation
Cornett W	Greenville Hospital System University Medical Center, Department of Surgery, Greenville, South Carolina 29605, USA. cschneider@ghs.org
Harper JL	Department of Radiation Oncology, Medical University of South Carolina, Charleston, SC 29425, USA. zauls@musc.edu
Pisano ED	Department of Radiology, Medical University of South Carolina College of Medicine, 96 Jonathan Lucas Street, Suite 601, MSC 617. Charleston, SC 29425, USA. pisanoe@musc.edu
Schneider C	Greenville Hospital System University Medical Center, Department of Surgery, Greenville, South Carolina 29605, USA. cschneider@ghs.org
Zauls AJ	Department of Radiation Oncology, Medical University of South Carolina, Charleston, SC 29425, USA. zauls@musc.edu

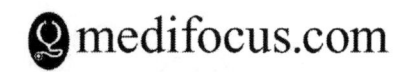

TN - Tennessee

Name of Author	Institutional Affiliation
Sanders ME	Department of Pathology, Vanderbilt University School of Medicine, Nashville, Tennessee 37232, USA.
Simpson JF	Department of Pathology, Vanderbilt University School of Medicine, Nashville, Tennessee 37232, USA.

TX - Texas

Name of Author	Institutional Affiliation
Arun B	Division of Cancer Medicine, The University of Texas M. D. Anderson Cancer Center, Houston, Texas, USA.
Babiera GV	Department of Surgical Oncology, The University of Texas MD Anderson Cancer Center, Houston, TX, USA.
Bailes AA	Department of Surgical Oncology, The University of Texas M. D. Anderson Cancer Center, Houston, USA.
Bayraktar S	Division of Cancer Medicine, The University of Texas M. D. Anderson Cancer Center, Houston, Texas, USA.
Beitsch P	Surgery, Dallas Breast Center, Dallas, TX, USA. Beitsch@aol.com
Beitsch PD	Department of Surgery, Dallas Breast Center, Dallas, TX, USA. beitsch@aol.com
Brewster AM	Department of Surgical Oncology, The University of Texas M. D. Anderson Cancer Center, Houston, USA.
Hunt KK	Department of Surgical Oncology, Unit 1484, The University of Texas MD Anderson Cancer Center, 1400 Pressler St, Houston, TX 77030, USA.
Kuerer HM	Department of Surgical Oncology, The University of Texas M. D. Anderson Cancer Center, Houston, TX, USA.
Lyden M	Department of Surgery, Dallas Breast Center, Dallas, TX, USA. beitsch@aol.com
Roses RE	Department of Surgical Oncology, The University of Texas M. D. Anderson Cancer Center, Houston, TX, USA.

Shaitelman SF	Department of Radiation Oncology, The University of Texas MD Anderson Cancer Center, Houston, Texas, USA.
Vicini FA	Department of Radiation Oncology, The University of Texas MD Anderson Cancer Center, Houston, Texas, USA.
Wagner JL	Department of Surgical Oncology, The University of Texas MD Anderson Cancer Center, Houston, TX, USA.
Yi M	Department of Surgical Oncology, Unit 1484, The University of Texas MD Anderson Cancer Center, 1400 Pressler St, Houston, TX 77030, USA.

UT - Utah

Name of Author	Institutional Affiliation
Cohen AL	Oncology Division, Department of Internal Medicine, University of Utah School of Medicine, Salt Lake City, Utah 84112-5550, USA.
Ward JH	Oncology Division, Department of Internal Medicine, University of Utah School of Medicine, Salt Lake City, Utah 84112-5550, USA.

VA - Virginia

Name of Author	Institutional Affiliation
Espina V	George Mason University, Center for Applied Proteomics and Molecular Medicine, Manassas, Virginia 20110, USA.
Liotta LA	George Mason University, Center for Applied Proteomics and Molecular Medicine, Manassas, Virginia 20110, USA.

WA - Washington

Name of Author	Institutional Affiliation
Lehman CD	Department of Radiology, University of Washington School of Medicine, Seattle Cancer Care Alliance, 825 Eastlake Ave E., G2-600, Seattle, WA 98109-1023, USA. lehman@u.washington.edu

Centers of Research

Other Countries

Australia

Name of Author	Institutional Affiliation
4Johnson CE	VBCRC Cancer Genetics Laboratory, Peter MacCallum Cancer Centre, Locked Bag 1, A'Beckett St, East Melbourne, Victoria, VIC 8006, Australia.
Davey C	Centre for Behavioural Research in Cancer, The Cancer Council Victoria, Carlton, Victoria, Australia.
De Morgan S	Faculty of Behavioural Science in Relation to Medicine, University of Newcastle, Newcastle, Australia. simoned@ihug.com.au
Dewey, Richard B Jr	VBCRC Cancer Genetics Laboratory, Peter MacCallum Cancer Centre, Locked Bag 1, A'Beckett St, East Melbourne, Victoria, VIC 8006, Australia.
Erbas B	Centre for Behavioural Research in Cancer, The Cancer Council Victoria, Carlton, Victoria, Australia.
Rogers K	Faculty of Behavioural Science in Relation to Medicine, University of Newcastle, Newcastle, Australia. simoned@ihug.com.au

Belgium

Name of Author	Institutional Affiliation
Altintas S	Department of Medical Oncology, Antwerp University Hospital, Edegem, Belgium. sevilay.altintas@uza.be
Sotiriou C	Department of Medical Oncology, Antwerp University Hospital, Edegem, Belgium. sevilay.altintas@uza.be

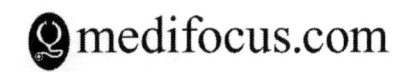

Canada

Name of Author	Institutional Affiliation
Bartlett JM	Ontario Institute for Cancer Research, Toronto, ON, Canada;
Diorio C	Oncology Research Unit, CHU de Quebec Research Centre, 1050 chemin Ste-Foy, Quebec City, QC, Canada, G1S 4L8. caroline.diorio@uresp.ulaval.ca.
Freeman CR	Division of Radiation Oncology, McGill University Health Centre, Montreal, QC, Canada.
Fyles AW	Radiation Medicine Program, Princess Margaret Hospital, Department of Radiation Oncology, University of Toronto, Canada M5G2M9.
Hathout L	Department of Radiation Oncology, Hopital Maisonneuve-Rosemont, Centre affilie a l'Universite de Montreal, Montreal, Quebec, Canada.
Hogue JC	Oncology Research Unit, CHU de Quebec Research Centre, 1050 chemin Ste-Foy, Quebec City, QC, Canada, G1S 4L8. caroline.diorio@uresp.ulaval.ca.
Lauzier S	Unite de recherche en sante des populations, Hopital du Saint-Sacrement, Centre de recherche du Centre hospitalier affile universitaire de Quebec, 1050 chemin Sainte-Foy, Quebec, QC, G1S 4L8, Canada.
Mesurolle B	1 All authors: Cedar Breast Clinic, McGill University Health Center, Royal Victoria Hospital, 687 Pine Ave W, Montreal, PQ, H3H 1A1 Canada.
Meterissian S	1 All authors: Cedar Breast Clinic, McGill University Health Center, Royal Victoria Hospital, 687 Pine Ave W, Montreal, PQ, H3H 1A1 Canada.
Olivotto IA	Radiation Therapy Program, BC Cancer Agency-Vancouver Island Centre, Victoria, BC, Canada. ewai@bccancer.bc.ca
Owen D	Radiation Therapy Program, Vancouver and Victoria, British Columbia, Canada.
Paszat L	Sunnybrook Health Sciences Centre, 2075 Bayview Avenue, Toronto, Ontario, Canada. Eileen.rakovitch@sunnybrook.ca

Provencher L	Unite de recherche en sante des populations, Hopital du Saint-Sacrement, Centre de recherche du Centre hospitalier affile universitaire de Quebec, 1050 chemin Sainte-Foy, Quebec, QC, G1S 4L8, Canada.
Rakovitch E	Sunnybrook Health Sciences Centre, 2075 Bayview Avenue, Toronto, Ontario, Canada. Eileen.rakovitch@sunnybrook.ca
Wai ES	Radiation Therapy Program, BC Cancer Agency-Vancouver Island Centre, Victoria, BC, Canada. ewai@bccancer.bc.ca
Williamson D	Radiation Medicine Program, Princess Margaret Hospital, Department of Radiation Oncology, University of Toronto, Canada M5G2M9.
Wong P	Division of Radiation Oncology, McGill University Health Centre, Montreal, QC, Canada.
Yassa M	Department of Radiation Oncology, Hopital Maisonneuve-Rosemont, Centre affilie a l'Universite de Montreal, Montreal, Quebec, Canada.

China

Name of Author	Institutional Affiliation
Li S	Breast Tumor Center, Sun Yat-Sen Memorial Hospital, 33 Yingfeng Road, Guangzhou, 510288, China.
Liao N	Southern Medical University, Guangzhou, China.
Su F	Breast Tumor Center, Sun Yat-Sen Memorial Hospital, 33 Yingfeng Road, Guangzhou, 510288, China.
Wu YL	Southern Medical University, Guangzhou, China.

Finland

Name of Author	Institutional Affiliation
Leidenius M	Helsinki University Central Hospital, Finland. elina.siponen@elisanet.fi
Leidenius MH	Breast Surgery Unit, Department of Gastrointestinal and General Surgery, Helsinki University Central Hospital, Helsinki, Finland. tuomo.meretoja@fimnet.fi

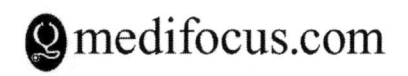

Meretoja TJ	Breast Surgery Unit, Department of Gastrointestinal and General Surgery, Helsinki University Central Hospital, Helsinki, Finland. tuomo.meretoja@fimnet.fi
Siponen E	Helsinki University Central Hospital, Finland. elina.siponen@elisanet.fi

France

Name of Author	Institutional Affiliation
Ansquer Y	Hopital St Antoine, Assistance Publique Hopitaux de Paris, Universite Pierre et Marie Curie, Paris VI, Service de Gynecologie Obstetrique, 184 rue du Faubourg St Antoine, 75012 Paris, Cedex 12, France. yan.ansquer@sat.aphp.fr
Avril A	Department of Surgery, Institut Bergonie, Bordeaux Cedex, France. tunon@bergonie.org
Bendifallah S	Department of Obstetrics and Gynecology, 4 Rue de la Chine, 75020 Paris, France. sofiane.bendifallah@yahoo.fr
Rouzier R	Department of Obstetrics and Gynecology, 4 Rue de la Chine, 75020 Paris, France. sofiane.bendifallah@yahoo.fr
Salmon R	Hopital St Antoine, Assistance Publique Hopitaux de Paris, Universite Pierre et Marie Curie, Paris VI, Service de Gynecologie Obstetrique, 184 rue du Faubourg St Antoine, 75012 Paris, Cedex 12, France. yan.ansquer@sat.aphp.fr
Tunon-de-Lara C	Department of Surgery, Institut Bergonie, Bordeaux Cedex, France. tunon@bergonie.org

Germany

Name of Author	Institutional Affiliation
Heil J	Breast Unit, University of Heidelberg Women's Hospital, Vossstrasse 9, 69115 Heidelberg, Germany.
Pantel K	Department of Gynaecology and Obstetrics, University Hospital Frankfurt, Frankfurt, Germany.
Rominger M	Klinik fur Strahlendiagnostik, Klinikum der Philipps-Univ. Marburg, Marburg, Germany. rominger@med.uni-marburg.de

Sanger N	Department of Gynaecology and Obstetrics, University Hospital Frankfurt, Frankfurt, Germany.
Schulz S	Breast Unit, University of Heidelberg Women's Hospital, Vossstrasse 9, 69115 Heidelberg, Germany.
Timmesfeld N	Klinik fur Strahlendiagnostik, Klinikum der Philipps-Univ. Marburg, Marburg, Germany. rominger@med.uni-marburg.de

Israel

Name of Author	Institutional Affiliation
Chikman B	Division of Surgery, Assaf Harofeh Medical Center, Zerifin, Israel. ahalevi@asaf.health.gov.il
Gutman M	Department of Diagnostic Imaging, Meir Medical Center, Kfar Saba, Israel.
Halevy A	Division of Surgery, Assaf Harofeh Medical Center, Zerifin, Israel. ahalevi@asaf.health.gov.il
Stackievicz R	Department of Diagnostic Imaging, Meir Medical Center, Kfar Saba, Israel.

Italy

Name of Author	Institutional Affiliation
Audisio R	Sandro Pitigliani Medical Oncology Unit, Istituto Toscano Tumori, Hospital of Prato, Prato, Italy. lbiganzoli@usl4.toscana.it
Barni S	Azienda Ospedaliera Treviglio-Caravaggio, BG, Italy. faupe@libero.it
Biganzoli L	Sandro Pitigliani Medical Oncology Unit, Istituto Toscano Tumori, Hospital of Prato, Prato, Italy. lbiganzoli@usl4.toscana.it
Biti G	Radiotherapy Unit, University of Florence, FLargo G. A. Brambilla 3, lorence, Italy. icro.meattini@unifi.it
Cassano E	Division of Breast Radiology, European Institute of Oncology, Via Ripamonti 435, Milan, Italy. chiara.trentin@ieo.it

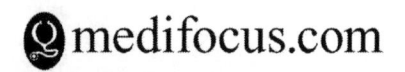

Cataliotti L	Breast Unit, University of Florence, Viale Morgagni 85, Florence, Italy. lorenzo.orzalesi@unifi.it
Cortesi L	Department of Oncology and Haematology, University of Modena and Reggio Emilia, Modena, Italy. hbc@unimore.it
Farante G	Division of Senology, European Institute of Oncology, IEO, Via Ripamonti 435, 20141 Milan, Italy. gabriel.farante@ieo.it
Federico M	Department of Oncology and Haematology, University of Modena and Reggio Emilia, Modena, Italy. hbc@unimore.it
Fozza A	Oncologia Radioterapica, IRCCS A.O.U. San Martino-IST-Istituto Nazionale per la Ricerca, sul Cancro, Largo R. Benzi, 10, 16132 Genoa, Italy. ale.fozza@libero.it
Guenzi M	Oncologia Radioterapica, IRCCS A.O.U. San Martino-IST-Istituto Nazionale per la Ricerca, sul Cancro, Largo R. Benzi, 10, 16132 Genoa, Italy. ale.fozza@libero.it
Meattini I	Radiotherapy Unit, University of Florence, FLargo G. A. Brambilla 3, lorence, Italy. icro.meattini@unifi.it
Orzalesi L	Breast Unit, University of Florence, Viale Morgagni 85, Florence, Italy. lorenzo.orzalesi@unifi.it
Petrelli F	Azienda Ospedaliera Treviglio-Caravaggio, BG, Italy. faupe@libero.it
Trentin C	Division of Breast Radiology, European Institute of Oncology, Via Ripamonti 435, Milan, Italy. chiara.trentin@ieo.it
Veronesi U	Division of Senology, European Institute of Oncology, IEO, Via Ripamonti 435, 20141 Milan, Italy. gabriel.farante@ieo.it

Japan

Name of Author	**Institutional Affiliation**
Akiyama F	Division of Pathology, The Cancer Institute of the Japanese Foundation for Cancer Research, Tokyo, Japan; Department of Pathology, The Cancer Institute Hospital of the Japanese Foundation for Cancer Research, Tokyo, Japan.

Iwase T	Department of Breast Surgery, Cancer Institute Hospital, Tokyo, Japan. ktada@jfcr.or.jp
Miyake T	Department of Breast and Endocrine Surgery, Osaka University, Graduate School of Medicine, Suita, Japan.
Miyashita M	Department of Surgery and Breast Surgery, Nihonkai General Hospital, 30 Akiho-cho, Sakata 998-8501, Japan. atihsayim8m8@med.tohoku.ac.jp
Noguchi S	Department of Breast and Endocrine Surgery, Osaka University, Graduate School of Medicine, Suita, Japan.
Ohuchi N	Department of Surgery and Breast Surgery, Nihonkai General Hospital, 30 Akiho-cho, Sakata 998-8501, Japan. atihsayim8m8@med.tohoku.ac.jp
Osako T	Division of Pathology, The Cancer Institute of the Japanese Foundation for Cancer Research, Tokyo, Japan; Department of Pathology, The Cancer Institute Hospital of the Japanese Foundation for Cancer Research, Tokyo, Japan.
Tada K	Department of Breast Surgery, Cancer Institute Hospital, Tokyo, Japan. ktada@jfcr.or.jp

Korea

Name of Author	Institutional Affiliation
6Ko BS	Department of Surgery, Asan Medical Center, University of Ulsan, College of Medicine, Seoul, Korea.
Hsiang HY.	Department of Surgery, Asan Medical Center, University of Ulsan, College of Medicine, Seoul, Korea.
Hwang SH	Breast Cancer Center, Department of Surgery, Gangnam Severance Hospital, Yonsei University College of Medicine, 211 Eonju-ro, Gangnam-gu, Seoul 135-720, Korea.
Kim J	Department of Surgery, Seoul National University College of Medicine, Seoul, Republic of Korea.
Lee HD	Breast Cancer Center, Department of Surgery, Gangnam Severance Hospital, Yonsei University College of Medicine, 211 Eonju-ro, Gangnam-gu, Seoul 135-720, Korea.

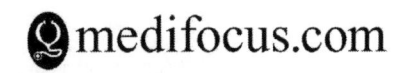

Noh DY	Department of Surgery, Seoul National University College of Medicine, Seoul, Republic of Korea.

Kuwait

Name of Author	Institutional Affiliation
Al Kandari F	Department of Nuclear Medicine, Hussain Makki Al Jumma Centre for Specialized Surgery, Khaitan, Kuwait. dr_shajji@yahoo.com
Usmani S	Department of Nuclear Medicine, Hussain Makki Al Jumma Centre for Specialized Surgery, Khaitan, Kuwait. dr_shajji@yahoo.com

Netherlands

Name of Author	Institutional Affiliation
Bijker N	Department of Radiotherapy, Academic Medical Centre, PO Box 22660, 1100 DD Amsterdam, the Netherlands. n.bijker@amc.uva.nl
Rutgers EJ	Department of Radiation Oncology, Academic Medical Center, P.O. Box 22700, 1100DE, Amsterdam, The Netherlands. n.bijker@amc.uva.nl
de Gelder R	Erasmus MC, Department of Public Health, P.O. Box 2040, 3000 CA, Rotterdam, The Netherlands. r.degelder@erasmusmc.nl
de Koning HJ	Erasmus MC, Department of Public Health, P.O. Box 2040, 3000 CA, Rotterdam, The Netherlands. r.degelder@erasmusmc.nl
van Tienhoven G	Department of Radiotherapy, Academic Medical Centre, PO Box 22660, 1100 DD Amsterdam, the Netherlands. n.bijker@amc.uva.nl

Singapore

Name of Author	Institutional Affiliation
Lim GH	Breast Department, KK Women's and Children's Hospital, Singapore, Singapore.
Liong YV	Breast Department, KK Women's and Children's Hospital, Singapore, Singapore.
Tan PH	Department of Radiation Oncology, National Cancer Centre Singapore, Singapore. Electronic address: fuhyong@yahoo.com.; Department of Radiation Oncology, National Cancer Centre Singapore, Singapore.; Department of Cancer Informatics, National Cancer Centre Singapore, Singapore.; Department of Radiation Oncology, National Cancer Centre Singapore, Singapore.; Department of Pathology, Singapore General Hospital, Singapore.
Thike AA	Department of Pathology, Singapore General Hospital, Singapore.
Wong FY	Department of Radiation Oncology, National Cancer Centre Singapore, Singapore. Electronic address: fuhyong@yahoo.com.; Department of Radiation Oncology, National Cancer Centre Singapore, Singapore.; Department of Cancer Informatics, National Cancer Centre Singapore, Singapore.; Department of Radiation Oncology, National Cancer Centre Singapore, Singapore.; Department of Pathology, Singapore General Hospital, Singapore.

Slovakia

Name of Author	Institutional Affiliation
Bartova M	IInd Department of Gynaecology and Obstetrics, University Hospital, Bratislava, Slovakia.
Pohlodek K	IInd Department of Gynaecology and Obstetrics, University Hospital, Bratislava, Slovakia.

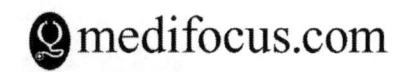

South Korea

Name of Author	Institutional Affiliation
Lee SK	Division of Breast and Endocrine Surgery, Department of Surgery, Samsung Medical Centre, Sungkyunkwan University School of Medicine, Seoul, South Korea.
Nam SJ	Division of Breast and Endocrine Surgery, Department of Surgery, Samsung Medical Centre, Sungkyunkwan University School of Medicine, Seoul, South Korea.

Spain

Name of Author	Institutional Affiliation
Estevez LG	Centro Integral Oncologico Clara Campal, Madrid, Spain. lauraestevez@hospitaldemadrid.com
Tusquets I	Centro Integral Oncologico Clara Campal, Madrid, Spain. lauraestevez@hospitaldemadrid.com

Sweden

Name of Author	Institutional Affiliation
Brandberg Y	Department of Molecular Medicine and Surgery, Karolinska Institutet, Karolinska University Hospital, P9:03, 171 76 Stockholm, Sweden. helena.sackey@ki.se
Sackey H	Department of Molecular Medicine and Surgery, Karolinska Institutet, Karolinska University Hospital, P9:03, 171 76 Stockholm, Sweden. helena.sackey@ki.se
Warnberg F	Department of Surgical Science, Uppsala University, Uppsala, SE-75105, Sweden. wenjing.zhou@surgsci.uu.se
Zetterlund L	Department of Surgery, Stockholm South General Hospital, Stockholm, Sweden; Department of Clinical Science and Education, Karolinska Institute, Stockholm, Sweden.
Zhou W	Department of Surgical Science, Uppsala University, Uppsala, SE-75105, Sweden. wenjing.zhou@surgsci.uu.se

de Boniface J	Department of Surgery, Stockholm South General Hospital, Stockholm, Sweden; Department of Clinical Science and Education, Karolinska Institute, Stockholm, Sweden.

Thailand

Name of Author	Institutional Affiliation
Raiyawa T	Division of Therapeutic Radiology and Oncology, Department of Radiology, Faculty of Medicine, Chulalongkorn University, Bangkok, Thailand.
Saksornchai K	Division of Therapeutic Radiology and Oncology, Department of Radiology, Faculty of Medicine, Chulalongkorn University, Bangkok, Thailand.

United Kingdom

Name of Author	Institutional Affiliation
Barnes NL	Array 2nd Floor, Education and Research Centre, Southmoor Road, Manchester M23 9LT, UK.
Benson JR	Cambridge Breast Unit, Addenbrooke's Hospital, Cambridge, UK; Anglia Ruskin University, Cambridge, UK. john.benson@addenbrookes.nhs.uk
Beral V	University of Oxford, Oxford, UK. gill.reeves@ceu.ox.ac.uk
Bruce J	Northumbria Healthcare NHS Foundation Trust, North Tyneside General Hospital, North Shields, UK.
Bundred NJ	Array 2nd Floor, Education and Research Centre, Southmoor Road, Manchester M23 9LT, UK.
Clark SE	Centre for Tumour Biology, Institute of Cancer and CR-UK Clinical Centre, Barts and the London School of Medicine and Dentistry, John Vane Science Centre, Charterhouse Square, London EC1M 6BQ, UK. sarahclark74@hotmail.com
Cuzick J	Cancer Research UK, Centre for Epidemiology, Mathematics, and Statistics, Wolfson Institute of Preventive Medicine, Queen Mary School of Medicine and Dentistry, University of London, London, UK. j.cuzick@qmul.ac.uk

Evans A	Ninewells Hospital and Medical School, Dundee, Scotland, UK. a.z.evans@dundee.ac.uk
George WD	Cancer Research UK, Centre for Epidemiology, Mathematics, and Statistics, Wolfson Institute of Preventive Medicine, Queen Mary School of Medicine and Dentistry, University of London, London, UK. j.cuzick@qmul.ac.uk
Howell A	Array Italy.; Pirkanmaa Cancer Society, Tampere, Finland.; Genesis Breast Cancer Prevention Centre, Manchester, UK.
Jones JL	Centre for Tumour Biology, Institute of Cancer and CR-UK Clinical Centre, Barts and the London School of Medicine and Dentistry, John Vane Science Centre, Charterhouse Square, London EC1M 6BQ, UK. sarahclark74@hotmail.com
Kennedy F	Sheffield Hallam University, UK. f.kennedy@shu.ac.uk
Lawrence GM	Cambridge Breast Unit and NIHR Cambridge Biomedical Research Unit, Box 97, Cambridge University Hospitals NHS Foundation Trust, Hills Road, Cambridge CB2 0QQ, UK. matthew.wallis@addenbrookes.nhs.uk
Mokbel K	The London Breast Institute, The Princess Grace Hospital, London, UK.
Pinder SE	Ninewells Hospital and Medical School, Dundee, Scotland, UK. a.z.evans@dundee.ac.uk
Reefy S	The London Breast Institute, The Princess Grace Hospital, London, UK.
Reeves GK	University of Oxford, Oxford, UK. gill.reeves@ceu.ox.ac.uk
Rumsey N	Sheffield Hallam University, UK. f.kennedy@shu.ac.uk
Staley H	Northumbria Healthcare NHS Foundation Trust, North Tyneside General Hospital, North Shields, UK.
Wallis MG	Cambridge Breast Unit and NIHR Cambridge Biomedical Research Unit, Box 97, Cambridge University Hospitals NHS Foundation Trust, Hills Road, Cambridge CB2 0QQ, UK. matthew.wallis@addenbrookes.nhs.uk
White P	Centre for Appearance Research, Faculty of Health and Life Sciences, University of the West of England, Bristol, United Kingdom. F.Kennedy@shu.ac.uk

Wishart GC — Cambridge Breast Unit, Addenbrooke's Hospital, Cambridge, UK; Anglia Ruskin University, Cambridge, UK. john.benson@addenbrookes.nhs.uk

NOTES

Use this page for taking notes as you review your Guidebook

5 - Tips on Finding and Choosing a Doctor

Introduction

One of the most important decisions confronting patients who have been diagnosed with a serious medical condition is finding and choosing a qualified physician who will deliver a high level and quality of medical care in accordance with currently accepted guidelines and standards of care. Finding the "best" doctor to manage your condition, however, can be a frustrating and time-consuming experience unless you know what you are looking for and how to go about finding it.

The process of finding and choosing a physician to manage your specific illness or condition is, in some respects, analogous to the process of making a decision about whether or not to invest in a particular stock or mutual fund. After all, you wouldn't invest your hard eared money in a stock or mutual fund without first doing exhaustive research about the stock or fund's past performance, current financial status, and projected future earnings. More than likely you would spend a considerable amount of time and energy doing your own research and consulting with your stock broker before making an informed decision about investing. The same general principle applies to the process of finding and choosing a physician. Although the process requires a considerable investment in terms of both time and energy, the potential payoff can be well worth it--after all, what can be more important than your health and well-being?

This section of your Guidebook offers important tips for how to find physicians as well as suggestions for how to make informed choices about choosing a doctor who is right for you.

Tips for Finding Physicians

Finding a highly qualified, competent, and compassionate physician to manage your specific illness or condition takes a lot of hard work and energy but is an investment that is well-worth the effort. It is important to keep in mind that you are not looking for just any general physician but rather for a physician who has expertise in the treatment and management of your specific illness or condition. Here are some suggestions for where you can turn to identify and locate physicians who specialize in managing your disorder:

medifocus.com

- **Your Doctor** - Your family physician (family medicine or internal medicine specialist) is a good starting point for finding a physician who specializes in your illness. Chances are that your doctor already knows several specialists in your geographic area who specialize in your illness and can recommend several names to you. Your doctor can also provide you with information about their qualifications, training, and hospital affiliations.

- **Your Peer Network** - Your family, friends, and co-workers can be a potentially very useful network for helping you find a physician who specializes in your illness. They may know someone else with this condition and may be able to put you in touch with them to find out which doctors they can recommend. If you have friends, neighbors, or relatives who work in hospitals (e.g., nurses, social workers, administrators), they may be a potentially valuable source for helping you find a physician who specializes in your condition.

- **Hospitals and Medical Centers** - Hospitals and medical centers are, potentially, an excellent source for finding physicians who specialize in treating specific diseases. Simply contact hospitals and major medical centers in your city, county, or state and ask if they have anyone on their staff who specializes in treating your condition. When you call, ask to speak to someone in the specific Department that cares for patients with the illness. For example, if you have been diagnosed with cancer, ask to speak with someone in the Department of Hematology and Oncology. If you are not sure which Department treats patients with your specific condition, ask to speak to someone in the Department of Medicine since this Department is the umbrella for many other medical specialties.

- **Organizations and Support Groups** - Many disease organizations and support groups that cater to patients with a specific illness or condition maintain physician referral lists and may be able to recommend doctors in your geographic area who specialize in the treatment and management of your specific disorder. This *MediFocus Guidebook* includes a select listing of disease organizations and support groups that you may wish to contact to ask for a physician referral.

- **Managed Care Plans** - If you belong to a managed care plan, you can obtain a list of physicians who belong to the Plan from the plan's membership services office. Keep in mind, however, that your choices will usually be limited to only those doctors who belong to the Plan. If you decide to go outside the Plan, you will likely have to pay for the doctor's services "out of pocket".

- **Medical Journals** - Many doctors based at major medical centers and universities who have special interest in a particular disease or condition conduct research and publish their findings in leading medical journals. Searching the medical literature can help you identify and locate leading physicians who are recognized as experts in their field about a particular illness. This *MediFocus Guidebook* includes an extensive listing of the names and institutional affiliations of physicians and researchers, in the United States and other countries, who have recently published their studies about this specific medical condition in leading medical journals. You can also conduct your own online search for your illness or condition and identify additional authors and hospitals who specialize in the disease using the PubMed database available at http://www.nlm.nih.gov.

- **American Medical Association** - The American Medical Association (AMA) is the nation's largest professional medical association that represents many doctors in the United States and also provides a free physician locator service called "AMA Physician Select" available at http://dbapps.ama-assn.org/aps/amahg.htm. You can search the AMA database by either "Physician Name" or "Medical Specialty". You can find information about physicians including medical school and residency training, area of specialty, and contact information.

- **American Board of Medical Specialists** - The American Board of Medical Specialists (ABMS) publishes a geographical list of board-certified physicians called the Official ABMS Directory of Board Certified Medical Specialists that is available in most public libraries. Physicians who are listed in the ABMS Directory are board-certified in a medical specialty meaning that they have passed rigorous certification examinations administered by a board of medical specialists. There are 24 specialty boards that are recognized by the ABMS and the AMA. Each candidate applying for board certification must pass a written examination given by the specific specialty board and 15 of the specialty boards also require candidates to pass an oral examination in order to obtain board certification. To find out if a particular physician you are considering is board certified:

    - Visit your local public library and ask for a copy of the Official ABMS Directory of Board Certified Medical Specialists.

    - Search the ABMS web site at http://www.abms.org/login.asp.

    - Call the ABMS toll free at 1-866-275-2267.

- **American Society of Clinical Oncology** - The American Society of Clinical Onclology (ASC)) is the largest professional organization that represents physicians who specialize in treating cancer patients (oncologists). The ASCO provides a searchable database of ASCO members called "Find an Oncologist" that you can access online at http://www.asco.org. You can search the "Find an Oncologist" database for a cancer specialist by name, city, state, country, or specialty area.

- **American Cancer Society** - The American Cancer Society (ACS) is a nationwide voluntary health organization dedicated to helping cancer patients and survivors through research, education, advocacy, and services. The ACS web site http://www.cancer.org is not only an excellent resource for cancer information but also includes a "Message Board" where you can ask questions, exchange ideas, and share stories. The ACS Message Board is also a potentially useful source for locating an oncologist in your geographical area who specializes in your specific type of cancer. You can also contact the ACS toll free by calling 1-800-ACS-2345.

- **National Comprehensive Cancer Network** - The National Comprehensive Cancer Network (NCCN) is an alliance of 19 of the world's leading cancer centers and is dedicated to helping patients and health care professionals make informed decisions about cancer care. You can find a listing of the 19 NCCN member cancer institutions on the NCCN web site at http://www.nccn.org/. You can also search the NCCN "Physician Directory" for doctors located at any of the 19 NCCN member cancer institutions at http://www.nccn.org/physician_directory/SearchPers.asp. This database is an excellent resource for locating leading cancer specialists nationwide who specialize in your specific type of cancer.

- **National Cancer Institute Clinical Trials Database** - The National Cancer Institute (NCI) is part of the National Institutes of Health (NIH) and coordinates the National Cancer Program which conducts and supports research, training, and a variety of other programs dedicated to prevention and treatment of cancer. The NCI maintains an extensive cancer clinical trials database that you can access at http://www.cancer.gov/clinicaltrials. You can search the database for current clinical trials by type of cancer and even limit your search to clinical trials within you geographical area by putting in your Zip Code. The NCI clinical trials database also provides contact information for the physicians who serve as the study coordinators for each clinical trial. This database is a valuable resource for identifying and locating leading physicians in your local area and around the country who are conducting cutting-edge clinical research about your specific type of cancer.

- **National Center for Complementary and Alternative Medicine** - The National Center for Complementary and Alternative Medicine (NCCAM) is part of the National Institutes of Health (NIH) and is dedicated to exploring complementary and alternative medicine healing practices in the context of rigorous scientific research and methodology. The NCCAM web site http://nccam.nih.gov/ includes publications, frequently asked questions, and useful links to other complementary and alternative medicine resources. If you have questions about complementary and alternative medicine practices for your particular illness or medical condition, you can contact the NCCAM Clearinghouse toll-free in the U.S. at 1-888-644-6226 or 301-519-3153. You can also contact the NCCAM Clearinghouse by E-mail: info@nccam.nih.gov.

- **National Organization for Rare Disorders** - The National Organization for Rare Disorders (NORD) is a federation of voluntary health organizations dedicated to helping patients with rare "orphan" diseases and their families. There are over 6,000 rare or "orphan" diseases that are estimated to affect approximately 25 million Americans. You can search NORD's "Rare Diseases Database" for information about rare diseases at http://www.rarediseases.org/search/rdblist.html. In addition to providing useful information about rare diseases, NORD maintains a confidential "Networking Program" for its members to enable them to communicate with other patients who suffer from the same disorder. To learn more about NORD's Networking Program, you can send an E mail to: orphan@rarediseases.org.

How to Make Informed Choices About Physicians

It has generally been assumed by many people that the longer a physician has been in practice, the more experience, knowledge, and skills he/she has accumulated and, therefore, the higher the quality of care they provide to their patients. Recent research conducted by a group of doctors from the Harvard Medical School, however, seems to strongly suggest that this premise may not be true. In an article published in February 2005 in the *Annals of Internal Medicine* (Volume 142, No. 4, pp. 260-303), the Harvard researchers seriously challenged the common assumption that the more clinical experience a physician has accumulated, the higher the level of medical care they provide to their patients.

In fact, surprisingly, the researchers found an inverse (opposite) relationship between the number of years that a physician has been in practice (i.e., experience) and the quality of care that the physician provides. In other words, the widely held belief that "practice makes perfect" does not necessarily apply to all physicians and should not be the sole criteria used by patients in their decision analysis for choosing a physician. The underlying message of this study is that the length of time a physician has been in practice does not necessarily equate to a high quality of medical care unless the doctor takes steps to keep abreast with new advances and changing patterns of clinical practice.

Here are some important issues you need to consider and carefully research before making an informed decision about choosing your doctor:

- **Board Certification** - Board certified doctors are required to have extra training after medical school to become specialists in a particular field of medicine and are required to take continuing education courses in order to maintain their board certification status. Check with the American Board of Medical Specialists (ABMS) to determine if a specific physician you are considering is board certified in a particular medical specialty. To find out if a particular physician you are considering is board certified:

  - Visit your local public library and ask for a copy of the Official ABMS Directory of Board Certified Medical Specialists.

  - Search the ABMS web site at http://www.abms.org/login.asp.

  - Call the ABMS toll free at 1-866-275-2267.

- **Experience** - As noted above, research from the Harvard Medical School strongly suggests that how long a physician has been in practice (i.e., experience) does not necessarily correlate with a high level of medical care. The most important issue, therefore, is not how long a doctor has been in practice but rather how much experience the physician has in treating your specific illness or medical condition. Some physicians who have been in practice for many decades may have only treated a small number of patients with the specific disorder, whereas, some younger physicians who have been in practice only a few years may have already treated hundreds of patients with the same disorder. Here are some suggestions for helping you find out about a particular physician's experience in treating your specific illness:

  - Call the physician's office and speak with a staff member such as a nurse or physician's assistant. Ask them for information about how many patients with your specific medical condition the physician treats during the course of a year. Ask how many patients with this condition the physician is currently treating. You will have to call several different physicians' offices in order to have a basis for comparing the numbers of patients.

  - Find out if the physician has published any articles about the condition in reputable medical journals by doing an author search online. You can conduct an online author search using PubMed at http://www.nlm.nih.gov. Simply click on the "PubMed" icon, select the "author" field from the "Limits" menu, enter the physician's name (last name followed by first initial), and then click on the "Go" button. The author search will retrieve all articles published by the particular physician you are considering.

- Talk with your family physician and ask if he/she can provide you with any information about the particular physician's experience in treating patients with your specific illness or condition.

- Contact disease organizations and support groups that specialize in helping patients with your specific disorder and ask if they can provide you with any information, including experience, about the physician you are considering.

- **Medical School Affiliation** - Find out if the physician you are considering also has a joint faculty appointment at a medical school. In general, practicing community physicians with a joint academic appointment at a medical school are more likely to be in contact with leading medical experts and may be more up-to-date with the latest advances in research and treatments than community based physicians who are not affiliated with a medical school.

- **Hospital Affiliation** - Find out about the hospitals that the doctor uses. In the event that you need to be treated at a hospital, is the hospital where the physician has admitting privileges nearby to your home or will you (and your family members) have to travel a considerable distance?

- **Hospital Accreditation** - Find out if the hospital where the physician has admitting privileges is accredited by the Joint Commission on Accreditation of Healthcare Organizations (JCAHO). You can find information about a specific hospital's accreditation status by searching the JCAHO web site at http://www.jointcommission.org/. The JCAHO is an independent, not-for-profit organization that evaluates and accredits more than 15,000 health care organizations and programs in the United States. To receive and maintain JCAHO accreditation, a health care organization must undergo an on-site survey by a JCAHO survey team at least every three years and meet specific standards and performance measurements that affect the safety and quality of patient care.

- **Health Insurance Coverage** - Find out if the physician is covered by your health insurance plan. If you belong to a managed care plan (HMO or PPO), you are usually restricted to using specific physicians who also belong to the Plan. If you decide to use a physician who is "outside the network," you will likely have to pay "out of pocket" for the services provided.

NOTES

Use this page for taking notes as you review your Guidebook

6 - Directory of Organizations

American Cancer Society
1599 Clifton Road, N.E.; Atlanta, GA, 30329
800.227.2345;   404.486.0100
www.cancer.org

American College of Obstetricians and Gynecologists
409 12th Street, SW; Washington, DC 20090-6920
202.638.5577
resources@acog.org
www.acog.org

American Institute for Cancer Research; Nutrition Hotline
1759 R St., NW.; Washington, DC 20009
800.843.8114;   202.328.7744
aicrweb@aicr.org
www.aicr.org

Breast Cancer Network of Strength
212 W. Van Buren Street; Suite 1000 Chicago, IL 60607-3908
800.221.2141;   312.986.8338
www.networkofstrength.org

BreastCancer.org
7 East Lancaster Avenue 3rd Floor Ardmore, PA 19003
www.breastcancer.org

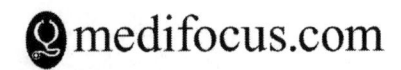

Cancer Care
275 Seventh Avenue; New York, NY 10001
800.813.4673; 212.712.8400
info@cancercare.org
www.cancercare.org

Cancer Caring Center
4117 Liberty Avenue; Pittsburgh, PA 15224
412.622.1212
info@cancercaring.org
www.cancercaring.org

Cancer Hope Network
2 North Road; Chester, NJ 07930
877.467.3638; 908.879.4039
info@cancerhopenetwork.org
www.cancerhopenetwork.org

Cancer Information Service; National Cancer Institute
6116 Executive Blvd.; Room 3036A; Bethesda, MD 20892
800.422.6237 800.332.8615 (TTY)
www.cancer.gov

CancerHelp (UK)
0808 800 40 40
www.cancerhelp.org.uk

Cleveland Clinic
9500 Euclid Avenue; Cleveland, OH 44221
800.223.2273; 216.444.2200;
www.ccf.org

Dana-Farber Cancer Institute
44 Binney Street; Boston, MA 02115
866.408.3324; 617.632.3000; 617.632.5530 (TDD)
www.dana-farber.org

Duke University Medical Center
Erwin Road Durham, NC 27710
(919) 684-8111
www.mc.duke.edu

European Organization for Research and Treatment of Cancer
Avenue E Mounier 83, boite 11; B-1200, Brussels; BELGIUM
+32 2-774-1611
www.eortc.be

Fox Chase Cancer Center
333 Cottman Avenue; Philadelphia, PA 19111
888.369.2427   215.728.6900
www.fccc.edu

H. Lee Moffitt Cancer Center and Research Institute
12902 Magnolia Drive Tampa, FL 33612
(813) 972-4673
www.moffitt.usf.edu

Hospital of the University of Pennsylvania
3400 Spruce Street Philadelphia, PA 19104
(215) 662-4000
www.pennhealth.com

Johns Hopkins Hospital
600 North Wolfe Street Baltimore, MD 21287
(410) 955-5000
www.hopkinsmedicine.org

Living Beyond Breast Cancer
354 West Lancaster Ave., Suite 224 Haverford, PA 19041
888.753.5222
www.lbbc.org

Look Good...Feel Better; American Cancer Society
1599 Clifton Road, NE; Atlanta, GA 30329
800.395.5665
www.lookgoodfeelbetter.org

M.D. Anderson Cancer Center
1515 Holcombe Blvd.; Houston, TX 77030
713.792.6161 713.792.3245; 800.392.1611
www.mdanderson.org

Macmillan Cancer Support; Cancer Backup
89 Albert Embankment London SE1 7UQ UK
020 7840 7840
www.macmillan.org.uk

Massachusetts General Hospital
55 Fruit Street Boston, MA 02114
(617) 726-2000
www.massgeneral.org

Mayo Clinic
1216 Second Street SW Rochester, MN 55902
(507) 255-5123
www.mayoclinic.org

Memorial Sloan-Kettering Cancer Center
1275 York Avenue; New York, NY 10021
800.525.2225 212.639.2000
www.mskcc.org

National Breast Cancer Foundation
2600 Network Blvd. Suite 300 Frisco, TX 75034
972.248.9200
www.nationalbreastcancer.org

National Comprehensive Cancer Network
275 Commerce Dr, Suite 300 Fort Washington, PA 19034
215.690.0300
www.nccn.org

National Lympedema Network
Latham Square 1611 Telegraph Avenue Suite 1111 Oakland, CA 94612
800.541.3259; 510.208.3200
nln@lymphnet.org
www.lymphnet.org

Ohio State University James Cancer Hospital
370 West 9th Avenue Columbus, OH 43210
(614) 293-8000
www.osumedcenter.edu

People Living with Cancer; American Society for Clinical Oncologists
2318 Mill Road, Suite 800, Alexandria, VA 22314
571-483-1780; 888-651-3038
www.cancer.net

Ronald Reagan UCLA Medical Center
10833 Le Conte Avenue Los Angeles, CA 90095
(310) 825-9111
www.uclahealth.org

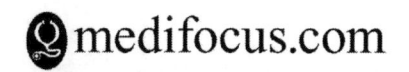

Rose Kushner Breast Cancer Advisory Center
POB 757; Malaga Cove, CA 90274
lkkushner@yahoo.com
www.rkbcac.org

SHARE: Self-Help for Women With Breast Cancer
1501 Broadway; Suite 704A; New York, NY 10036
866.891.2392; 212.719.0364
www.sharecancersupport.org

Stanford Hospital and Clinics
300 Pasteur Drive Palo Alto, CA 94304
(650) 723-4000
www.stanfordhospital.com

Susan G. Komen Breast Cancer Foundation
5005 LBJ Freeway, Suite 250; Dallas, TX 75244
877.465.6636
www.komen.org

The Breast Cancer Site
One Union Square 600 University Street Suite 1000 Seattle, WA 98101
www.thebreastcancersite.com

The Cancer Project; Cancer and Nutrition
5100 Wisconsin Avenue Suite 400 Washington, DC 20016
202.244.5038
www.cancerproject.org

medifocus.com

The Wellness Community
919 18th St. NW Suite 54 Washington, DC 20006
202.659.9709; 888.793.9355
www.thewellnesscommunity.org

University of Alabama Hospital
619 South 19th Street Birmingham, AL 35233
(205) 934-4011
www.health.uab.edu

University of California, San Francisco Medical Center
500 Parnassus Avenue San Francisco, CA 94143
(415) 476-1000
www.ucsfhealth.org

University of Chicago Hospital; Cancer Research Center
5841 South Maryland Avenue; Chicago, IL 60637
877.824.0660   773.702.1000
www.uchospitals.edu/specialties/cancer

University of Michigan Hospitals and Health Centers
1500 East Medical Center Drive Ann Arbor, MI 48109
(734) 936-4000
www.med.umich.edu

University of Washington Medical Center
1959 NE Pacific St, Box 356151 Seattle, WA 98195
(206) 598-3300
www.uwmedicine.org/Facilities/UWMedicalCenter/

Vanderbilt University Medical Center
1211 22nd Avenue South Nashville, TN 37232
(615) 322-5000
www.mc.vanderbilt.edu

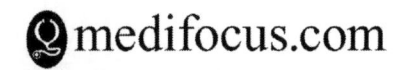

Women's Cancer Network; Gynecologic Cancer Foundation
230 W. Monroe; Suite 2528; Chicago, IL 60606
312.578.1439
info@thegcf.org
www.wcn.org

Women's Cancer Resource Center
5741 Telegraph Avenue; Oakland, CA 94609
888.421.7900; 510.420.7900
wcrc@wcrc.org
www.wcrc.org

Young Survival Coalition
61 Broadway, Suite 2235 New York, NY 10006
877-973-1011; 646-257-3000
www.youngsurvival.org/

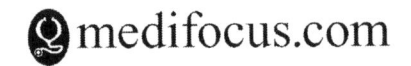

Complementary and Alternative Medicine Resources

American Academy of Medical Acupuncture
170 East Grand Avenue Suite 330 El Segundo, CA 90245 Phone: 310.364.0193
administrato@medicalacupuncture.org
http://www.medicalacupuncture.org

American Association for Acupuncture and Oriental Medicine
1925 West County Road B2
Roseville, MN 55113
Phone: 651.631.0216
http://www.aaaom.edu

American Association of Naturopathic Physicians
4435 Wisconsin Avenue
Suite 403 Washington, DC 20016
Phone (Toll free): 866.538.2267
Phone: 202.237.8150
http://www.naturopathic.org

American Chiropractic Association
1701 Clarendon Blvd.
Arlington, VA 22209
Phone: 703.276.8800 memberinfo@acatoday.org http://www.amerchiro.org

American Holistic Medical Association
23366 Commerce Park Suite 101B Beachwood, OH 44122 Phone: 216.292.6644
info@holisticmedicine.org http://www.holisticmedicine.org

American Massage Therapy Association
500 Davis Street, Suite 900
Evanston, IL 60201-4695
Phone (Toll-Free): 877.905.2700
Phone: 847.864.0123 info@amtamassage.org http://www.amtamassage.org

National Center for Complementary and Alternative Medicine (NCCAM) Clearinghouse
9000 Rockville Pike Bethesda, MD 20892 Phone: 888.644.6226 info@nccam.nih.gov

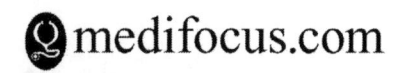

http://nccam.nih.gov

National Center for Homeopathy
801 North Fairfax Street, Suite 306
Alexandria, VA 22314
Phone: 703.548.7790
http://www.homeopathic.org

Office of Dietary Supplements, National Institutes of Health
6100 Executive Boulevard
Room 3B01, MSC 7517
Bethesda, MD 20892-7517
Phone: 301.435.2920   ods@nih.gov   http://ods.od.nih.gov

Rosenthal Center for Complementary and Alternative Medicine
Columbia Presbyterian Hospital
630 West 168th Street
Box 75
New York, NY 10032
Phone: 212.342.0101
http://rosenthal.hs.columbia.edu

Made in the USA
Lexington, KY
03 August 2016